HOW TO BE
a Redhead

A Guide to Beauty, Skincare, Hair Care, Fashion and Confidence
From the Sisters Who Started the Red Hair Revolution

Adrienne & Stephanie Vendetti

creators of How to be a Redhead

PAGE STREET
PUBLISHING CO.

PAGE STREET
PUBLISHING CO.

Copyright © 2016 Adrienne & Stephanie Vendetti

First published in 2016 by
Page Street Publishing Co.
27 Congress Street, Suite 103
Salem, MA 01970
www.pagestreetpublishing.com

All rights reserved. No part of this book may be reproduced or used, in any form or by any means, electronic or mechanical, without prior permission in writing from the publisher.

Distributed by Macmillan, sales in Canada by The Canadian Manda Group.

19   18   17   16   1   2   3   4   5

ISBN-13: 978-1-62414-222-2
ISBN-10: 1-62414-222-2

Library of Congress Control Number: 2015948492

Cover and book design by Page Street Publishing Co.
Photography by Luciana Pampalone
Illustrations by Ekaterina Petropavlovskaia (kateillustrate) & Yarden Karako

Printed and bound in China

Page Street is proud to be a member of 1% for the Planet. Members donate one percent of their sales to one or more of the over 1,500 environmental and sustainability charities across the globe who participate in this program.

For our redhead grandmother, Rosemary Vendetti, for teaching us
How to be a Redhead.

For our parents, for always teaching us to think big and for always
supporting us.

For our husbands, for believing in our dreams.

And most of all, for our followers, whom we call our "redhead beauties;"
we wouldn't be anywhere without you!

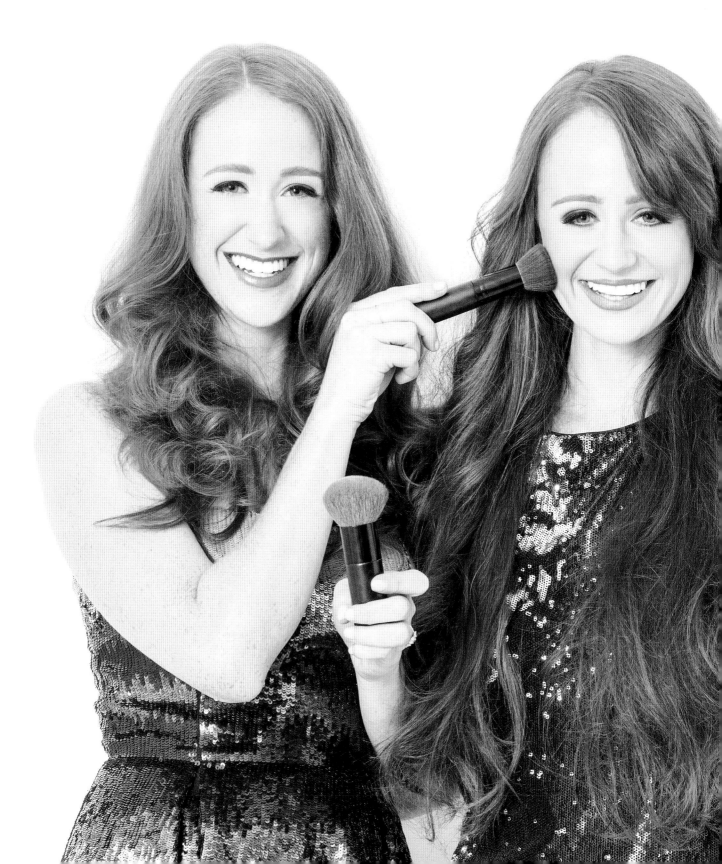

contents

what people are saying about our site

"Through How to be a Redhead, she found a good organic sunscreen and a foundation, plus the confidence to wear scarlet lipstick, a shade she had always thought was off limits." —*The New York Times*

"Growing up, sisters Adrienne and Stephanie Vendetti say they were always searching for hair and makeup products that would suit their cinnamon tresses and alabaster complexions. But despite redheads making up 6% of the U.S. population, the women felt mostly ignored by mainstream beauty magazines and websites. So, after years of toying around with the idea, they decided to start their own." —ABC News

"After testing hundreds of beauty products, the sisters decided to start a website to share their redhead know-how." —*SHAPE* magazine

"Clearly, there was a gaping hole in the market, but since How to be a Redhead's inception (or was it its influence?) many makeup companies carry shades that flatter more than just blondes and brunettes." —Refinery29

"[S]isters have turned their experiences into the largest redhead-focused beauty site in America." —*Daily Mail*

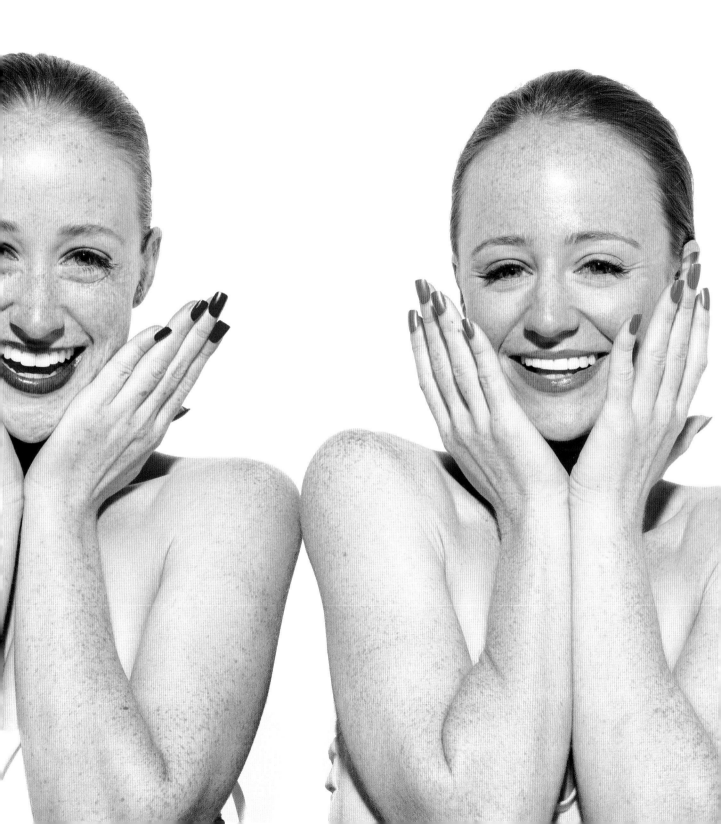

our story

We grew up in a small town in Rhode Island and were the only two redheads in our school. Being two years apart, we were always close friends and from an early age loved to experiment with beauty products. Unlike our friends at school, our eyelashes were blonde, our skin was fair and our hair was vibrantly red. When friends would share their favorite lip gloss, mascara or lotion, we knew our coloring and sensitive skin required its own "redhead friendly" products. We have fond memories of testing hundreds of products together in our home bathroom, and always joked that we knew How to be a Redhead. The name stuck and never left us.

Fast-forward to college and we were both studying business at the University of Miami. We would spend countless hours discussing how we should write a book about How to be a Redhead. Websites weren't as popular as they are now, and we figured we would put all of our knowledge of redhead beauty into one book. We always envisioned having a space where redheads could go to and feel trendy, while getting the best beauty and fashion advice. The goal was to have a redhead's blonde and brunette friends and family say, "Being a redhead is so cool! I want to have red hair."

We decided to start the How to be a Redhead blog. Our aim was to empower every redhead woman to feel confident, look amazing and rock her beauty. We are strong believers in our catch phrase: Red hair is more than a hair color, it's a lifestyle!

Within six months, we grew the blog into a website, and soon, How to be a Redhead became our full-time job. Shortly thereafter, we moved into a tiny apartment in the Upper West Side of New York City and worked tirelessly to accomplish years of vision. Since, we've grown How to be a Redhead to the brand it is now and have been featured in the biggest publications in the world. It is now our life mission to empower redheads around the world to rock it like a redhead with pure confidence.

So, here we are. *Wow!* The *How to be a Redhead* book is here, and it's truly a dream come true. To make it even more exciting, this is the first beauty book dedicated to redheads. It's incredible that we are able to give you all a voice in the beauty and fashion community. There is not a minute that goes by that we do not thank our followers, whom we call our "redhead beauties." We couldn't do any of this without you. Your tweets, messages, emails and comments have truly given us the confidence to rock our red hair too. We hope this book provides you with the best beauty and fashion tips for your redhead life, but most of all we hope it gives you the confidence to live a beautiful life. We hope this new platform genuinely gives all redheads an inner strength they never knew they had.

This book is making history and we are doing it together, as one beautiful community. We would not have it any other way.

Rock it like a Redhead!

Love,
Adrienne & Stephanie

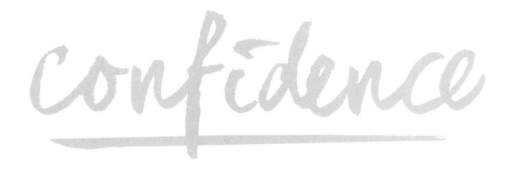

confidence

"I love that our hair isn't simply a color,
but a real identity. One of my favorite things is to
pass another natural redhead on the street, and do that
little acknowledgement thing that redheads do—a small
nod, a tiny smile—we're proud and we cheer each other
on. Being a redhead means that I get to be a magical
unicorn. I'm part of the small population that naturally has
this gorgeous color, and that makes me (and my
fellow gingers) so incredibly unique."

—Erin La Rosa, redhead and
BuzzFeed deputy editorial director

This book will provide you with the best advice and tips for redheads, but confidence is the first step to true beauty. Since the whole world admires the beauty of red hair, redheads should feel empowered by its distinctiveness. We define "redhead confidence" as the ability to love, embrace and accept your red hair and unique features.

In most cases, a redhead is usually the only person with red hair in a room and it can be tough to stand out when all one wants to do (especially during the teenage years) is fit in. There are many mean nicknames and phrases used to describe a redhead's presence, and many call these acts "ginger bullying" or "redhead bullying." We're overjoyed when we hear from our followers that HowtoBeaRedhead.com has served as a positive place for redheads to feel confident enough to go to school or work. We hope this book will do the same for you.

Redheads can choose to let bullies bother them, or they can hold their head high and respond with, "I know, isn't my hair amazing?" It took us years to figure out this secret. Going into a shell the minute someone calls you ginger, carrot top and/or strawberry will only make situations worse. We always suggest to "fake it until you feel it" or to genuinely respond with a confidence-boosting response.

If you're a redhead experiencing bullying, do know that it will pass. There will be a sudden shift when everyone begins to compliment and love your red locks (for us, it was in college). It goes from, "Go away, carrot top" to "Your hair is absolutely stunning." Children can be mean, but always know that people are envious of red hair because it is the most gorgeous hair color in the world.

Keep your head high and rock that red hair with pure confidence.

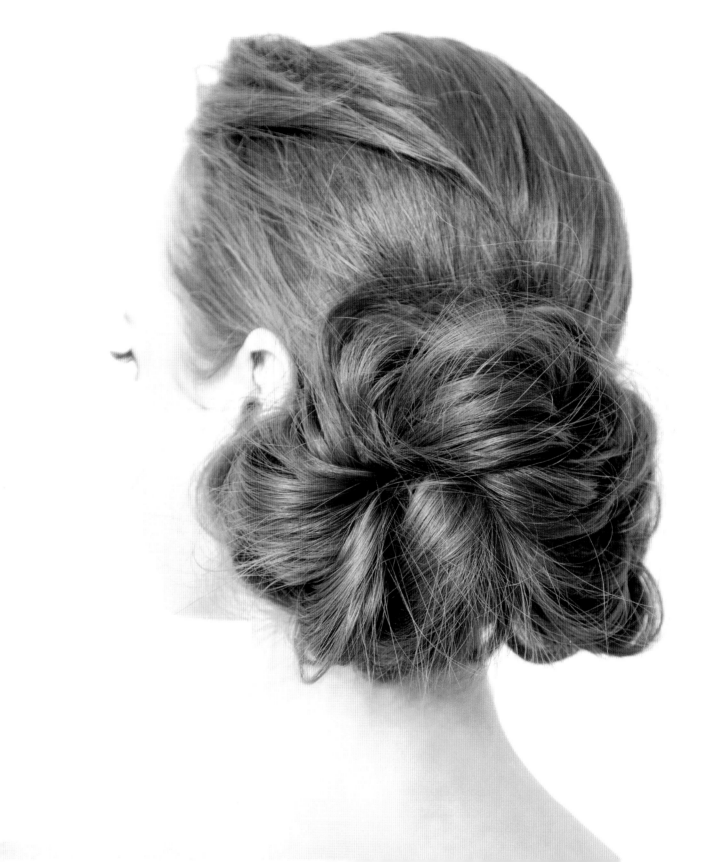

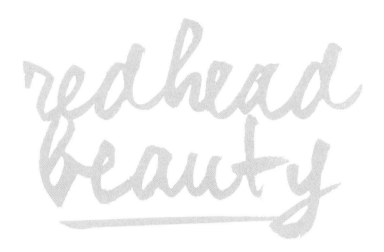

our "redhead friendly" approval process

We always thought it would be wonderful (and informative) to have products marked "redhead friendly" when purchasing them at a drugstore or local department store. That way, redheads save hundreds of dollars on unused products and know immediately that the product will work for them.

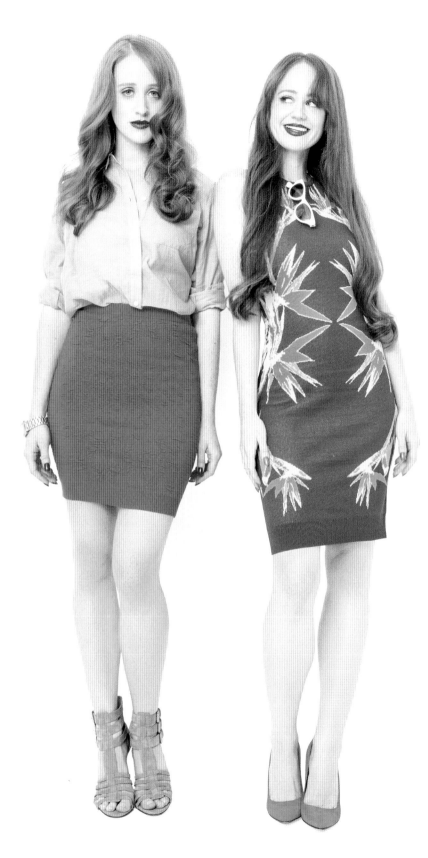

We apply the same concept in this very book. All brands and products mentioned have been tested on a redhead for a maximum of ten days. If it passes, it is deemed "redhead friendly," meaning a redhead can trust that the product works for her skin and/or hair. If it fails, it means one of the following things happened:

1. It made the skin break out.

2. It irritated sensitive skin.

3. The item did not complement red hair or particular skin tones.

4. The products had an excess of harsh chemicals.

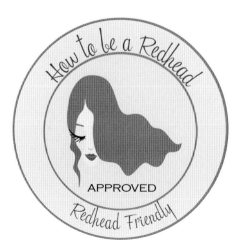

How to be a Redhead
APPROVED
Redhead Friendly

five steps for "redhead friendly" products

1

We search for products that complement a redhead. All beauty products must be designed to complement sensitive, fair skin and red hair. They must be made without harsh chemicals.

2

Companies send their products to the How to be a Redhead team for approval.

3

Product is then tried for a maximum of ten days by a natural redhead.

4

If the product does not cause irritation or harm the hair or skin in any way, the item is then deemed "redhead friendly" and receives the stamp of approval.

5

How to be a Redhead will then work with the company to spread the news about the product to the redhead community.

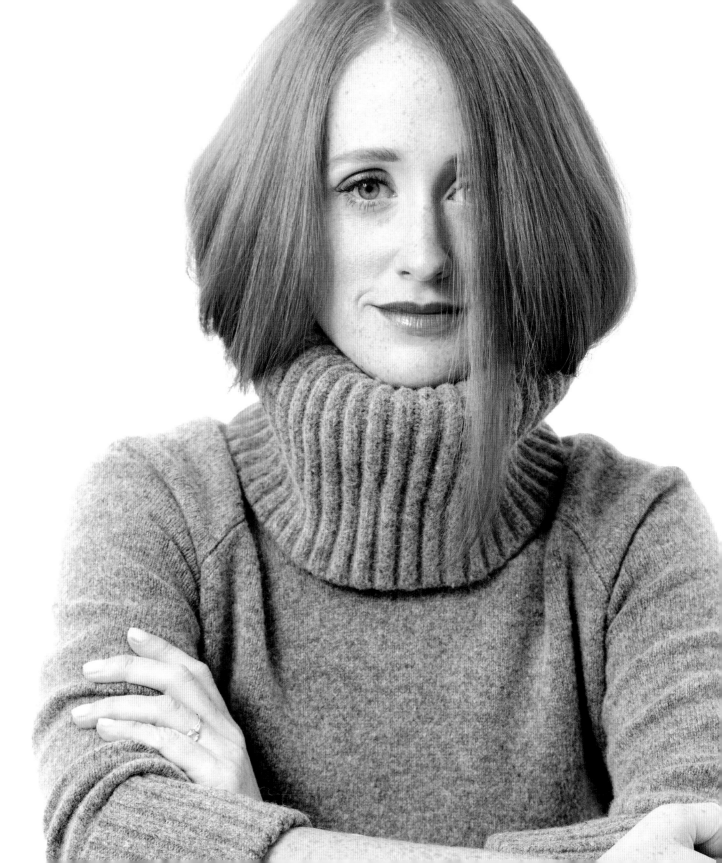

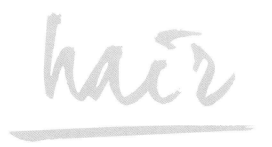

"Color connects with our emotions. In life,
when we see color it affects our feelings.
Red can be associated with hot, and redheads
are thought to be a fiery breed."

-Nick Arrojo, owner & founder of ARROJO NYC

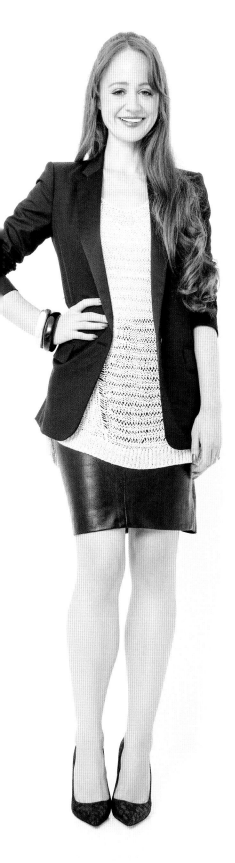

Hair is a huge part of a redhead's identity, not only because the color is unique, but also because it defines a person. People recognize a redhead from miles away and commonly describe them as "the one with red hair." If you were anything like us growing up, your red hair was probably (as our mom described it) uncontrollable. In our later years, we learned that the uncontrollable nature of our hair had a strong connection with our feisty personalities. But we'll save that for later.

For a redhead, hair is everything because the color itself is attention grabbing. It screams, "Look at me!" This is why redheads are under the most pressure to keep their locks looking gorgeous.

Adrienne has a wild, frizzy and coarse mane, but with strong natural color. Stephanie has wavy locks and struggles to keep the red vibrant enough. Throughout the years, we have mastered how to make red hair look great with certain tips, suggestions and "redhead friendly" beauty products.

Definition of a natural redhead: someone born with red hair.

"An exotic woman with a fiery temper.
One of the most beautiful creatures on Earth,
too bad there are so little of them. Redheads are
commonly a human, characterized by pale skin,
freckles and bright red hair."

—Urban Dictionary

Definition of a "by choice" redhead: someone who dyes their hair red.

the different red hair colors

Red hair is categorized as light, medium or dark. Within those shades there are different tones, defined as the following:

cool toned

Hair that is on the lighter side and usually lacks warmth.

strawberry: This is the subtlest of the reds. It is a cheerful blend of blonde with earthy red that makes a beautiful version any redhead should be proud to wear.

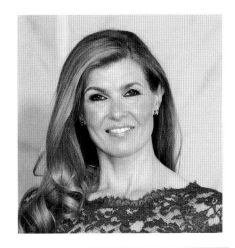

copper: This color is also known as ginger. The shade is sometimes mistaken for more orange than red. This tone falls somewhere between strawberry and the classic red. It has more orange in it than the subtler strawberry and less red than classic red.

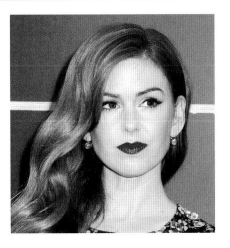

warm toned

Hair that is on the warm side, with rich undertones.

classic red: This is the red often imagined when people picture a redhead. It is vibrant, deep and attention grabbing. This red is richer than almost any other hair color.

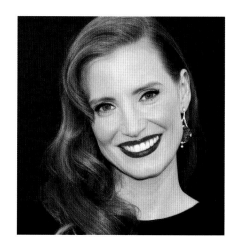

deep red: Darker than the classic red. This color is a gentler version of the auburn tone; it has all of the rich darkness and hints of brown.

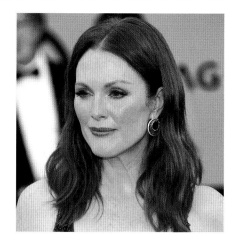

Natural redheads do not turn gray like blondes and brunettes do. Red hair initially tends to turn blonde and then white.

Just like fingerprints, no one has identical shades of red hair. This applies to natural and "by choice" redheads. Redheads should be proud of their unique, imprinted code.

auburn: The darker side of the red family. This color verges on being defined as brown, but luckily, it easily holds enough red to ensure the person is a redhead. The red tones bring a vitality and joy to the shade.

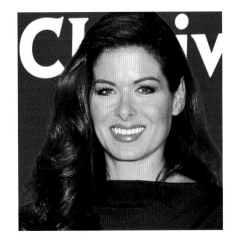

deep auburn: This is a rich and deep tone of red hair with more hints of brown than red.

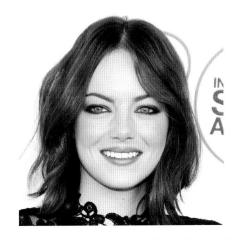

red violet: Just like strawberry blonde, this color is sometimes mistaken as not being in the red family. It's absolutely a version of red and is the deepest of them all.

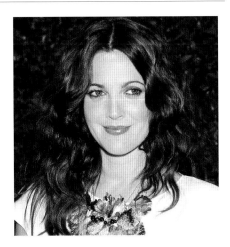

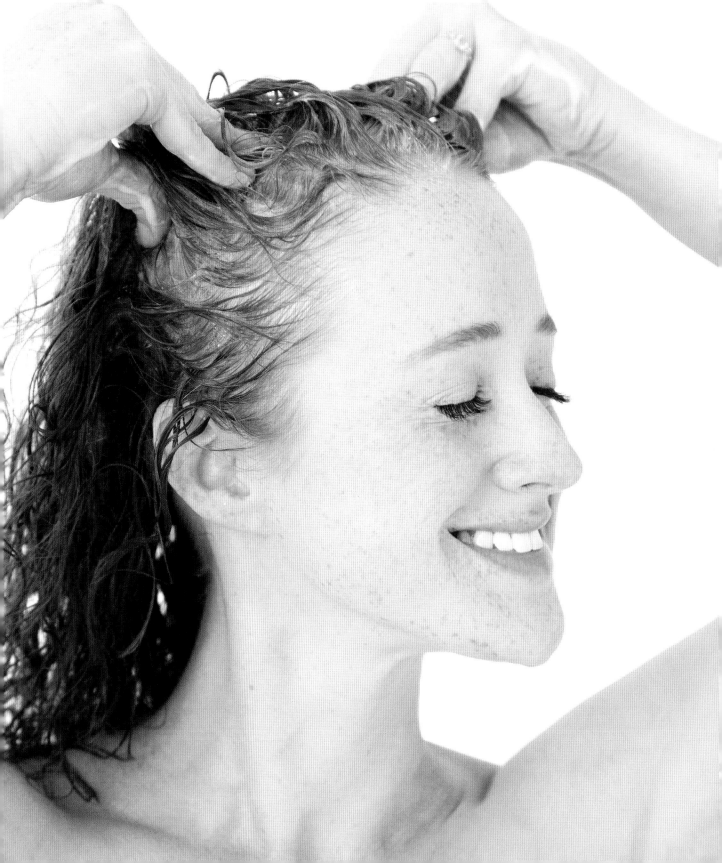

how to prep red hair
the best shampoo & conditioners
for your hair type

We began experimenting with different hair products when we were in middle school. We vividly remember scouting through aisles at big-name stores to find the perfect shampoo and conditioners. We'd buy and test different brands to see which worked the best with our red hair. It was noticeable almost immediately that the products with heavy chemicals made our hair felt soft at first, but days later, our hair was frizzier and seemed angry with us. *It's true!* Hair has a temper (especially RED hair) and wants to be treated with care. That's when we realized that sulfate-free and paraben-free products were best for redheads.

Redheads, either natural or by choice, should always choose sulfate-free and paraben-free shampoos and conditioners. Chemicals can strip the hair and create breakage, and they can even dull color (whether you're natural or by choice). If you want to go a step further, 100% natural hair products with absolutely zero chemicals are an even better choice as they provide superior results. The more natural, the better!

A sulfate-free shampoo is a shampoo that does not contain sodium lauryl sulfate (SLS). Parabens are preservatives that prevent bacterial growth, used in many different products because they are inexpensive and effective. Also, products with sulfates and parabens can stay on shelves longer. The chemicals in both sulfates and parabens can irritate the scalp, excessively strip essential oils and cause hair to dry out.

do you have a dry, oily or normal scalp?

(1)

dry hair

This is the most common hair type among redheads. Adrienne has this hair type, and it is the exact reason why she does not wash her hair frequently. Dry hair is coarse, unruly and shows signs of damage such as split ends and breakage. It's caused by a lack of natural oils produced by your scalp to keep your hair soft.

best dandruff shampoo/conditioner for your red hair

$: AVEENO ® NOURISH+ DANDRUFF CONTROL shampoo and conditioner

$$: Max Green Alchemy Scalp Rescue Shampoo and Conditioner

Dandruff is the most common scalp condition among redheads with sensitive skin, dry and/or oily hair. The yellow or white flakes at the top of the hairline are actually dead skin. Choose a gentle shampoo and conditioner that will not cause irritation.

Tip: Bacteria can live in hats, so just like all other clothing, they must be laundered to prevent bacteria from returning and causing the reoccurrence of dandruff.

"Because redheads are usually a little more sensitive to product ingredients, be careful when selecting products to combat oily scalps. Number one reason people have a perpetually oily scalp is over cleansing. If you do shampoo daily as you may have an oilier scalp than most, choose a shampoo that doesn't contain a chemical solvent."

—Christyn M. Nawrot, redhead & national training director
of PHYTO HAIR CARE

2

oily hair

Excessive oil production by glands in the scalp can be a problematic condition causing greasy hair and dandruff.

3

combination/normal hair

A happy medium. Stephanie has this hair type, and depending on the season, has a mixture of dry and oily locks.

red hair types

straight hair

This type of hair is straight and next to impossible to curl. It is commonly the most oily hair type.

wavy hair

Hair that is somewhere between straight and curly. This hair type is prone to frizz, but not as much as curly hair is.

curly hair

Curly hair has a definite *S* shape, with or without products. This hair type is usually full-bodied and prone to frizziness and damage. Curly hair requires the most maintenance and if not properly taken care of can result in dull-looking hair.

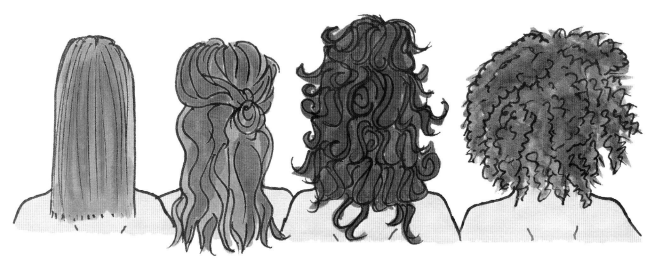

kinky hair

This hair type is tightly coiled and very fragile. Instead of an "S" shape, the hair type has a zigzag pattern. This is the driest hair type. It is prone to breakage and requires a gentle touch. Experts recommend treating this hair type like a fine silk blouse: cleanse gently, detangle softly and avoid harsh chemicals.

red hair textures

1

fine hair

Fine hair happens when each individual strand is thin. It is the most fragile hair and requires the most care because it can be easily damaged. It is a fact that people with finer hair tend to have more hair than people with thicker strands. Fine hair can be oilier than other hair types because the fine texture of the hair absorbs oil very easily. For this reason, redheads with fine hair should learn how to style hair correctly. This hair type usually can't hold styles well, but certain products can help you get the look you desire.

best "redhead friendly" products for thinning hair

$: OGX Biotin & Collagen shampoo and conditioner

$$: Keranique Scalp Stimulating shampoo and conditioner

Fellow redhead and national training director of PHYTO Hair Care, Christyn M. Nawrot gives us the scoop on thinning hair:

Thinning hair is definitely different from fine hair. Everyone has a genetic predisposition to have fine, medium or thick hair, just as we are predisposed to have a certain hair color. If you're born with fine hair you're probably going to have smaller hair density, meaning a smaller diameter of each strand of hair on your head.

More times than not, the (genetic) color of your hair determines how much hair you have per square inch. Blondes usually have the most hair per square inch, followed by redheads, and the darker the hair becomes the less hair they usually have. But thinning hair is not more predisposed due to your natural hair color. Redheads are subject to the same variables and causes of thinning hair as any other natural color of hair. Thinning hair is not always a direct result of having fine hair either. The main contribution for thinning hair is a disrupted growth cycle.

Thinning hair happens when the growth cycles are compromised due to changes in the phases of growth. The anagen phase (active growth phase) is shortened, prolonging your catagen phase (resting phase) and the telogen phase (falling out phase) is significantly lengthened, causing the hair to thin. There are three main types of hair thinning:

1. TEMPORARY HAIR THINNING is caused by stress, medication, diet, fatigue, hormones and seasonal changes that can cause premature hair thinning. Phytocyane and phytogrowth both work to counteract temporary thinning.

2. TRACTION HAIR THINNING is caused by braiding, weaving, extensions and excessive heat styling (such as blow drying, curling and straightening). These factors cause collagen to build up around the hair follicle, preventing healthy, new hair growth. This can then lead to hair thinning. Phytotraxil works to counteract traction hair thinning.

3. CHRONIC AND SEVERE HAIR THINNING is caused by a genetic predisposition for premature hair thinning. Phytolium 4 works to counteract chronic and severe hair thinning.

Yet, a healthy diet, plenty of sleep and sufficient exercise and physical activity are always going to positively regulate the body. Also, stay away from hair products that contain heavy waxes and silicones that coat and clog the scalp. Many of these products are notorious for causing dormancy in the hair growth cycles that can ultimately contribute to hair thinning. Regular scalp massaging, at least once a week, with a natural fiber boar bristle brush to gently stimulate the scalp is always a good idea to promote microcirculation without injuring the scalp.

coarse hair

Many people think that if you have coarse hair, you also have curly hair. This is a common misconception. In fact, most redheads have coarse hair and can also have a combination of thin, straight, wavy, frizzy and/or curly hair. If you have this hair type, the hair is actually thicker. When coarse hair is properly cared for, it can be soft and silky. If your hair is rough to the touch, your hair is probably dry or damaged. It does take effort to get it to shine, which is why we recommend using minimal heat products and the proper "redhead friendly" products.

frizzy hair

Common among wavy, curly and kinky hair types, frizzy hair occurs when moisture passes through the hair and the strands swell. As a result, hair appears dry and frizzy.

Because redheads have thicker hair than people with other hair colors, they have fewer strands of hair. For example, while blondes have on average 140,000 hairs, redheads have approximately 90,000, according to Cass Cort's *The Redhead Handbook*.

natural redheads

the best shampoos + conditioners for hair type

For "by choice" redheads, turn to page 71 for shampoo recommendations. All redheads can use these shampoos, but certain "color enhancing" products are best for vibrancy.

	normal This hair type is commonly normal, not dry or oily	fine This hair type is commonly oily	coarse This hair type is commonly dry	frizzy This hair type is commonly dry
straight	$: OGX Brazilian Keratin Therapy Shampoo $$: John Masters Organics Lavender Rosemary Shampoo for Normal Hair and Citrus & Neroli Detangler	$: Giovanni Tea Tree Triple Treat Shampoo + Conditioner $$: Bumble + Bumble Thickening Shampoo and Conditioner	$: Alba Botanica Drink It Up Coconut Milk Shampoo + Conditioner $$: SHU UEMURA Moisture Velvet Nourishing Shampoo + Conditioner	$: Avalon Organics Smoothing Grapefruit & Geranium Shampoo + Conditioner $$: ALETERNA Haircare Bamboo Smooth Anti-Frizz Shampoo + Conditioner
wavy	$: ARROJO Gentle Shampoo + Conditioner $$: Oribe Signature Shampoo + Conditioner	$: Aveeno Pure Renewal Shampoo + Conditioner $$: Moroccanoil Extra Volume Shampoo + Conditioner	$: Wella Brilliance Shampoo & Conditioner For Coarse Hair $$: Fekkai Essential Shea Shampoo & Conditioner	$: Acure Organics Moroccan Argan Oil + Argan Stem Cell Shampoo + Conditioner $$: Klorane Shampoo + Conditioner with Papyrus Milk

	normal	fine	coarse	frizzy
	This hair type is commonly normal, not dry or oily	This hair type is commonly oily	This hair type is commonly dry	This hair type is commonly dry
curly	$: Marc Anthony Curl Defining Shampoo + Conditioner $$: DevaCurl No-Poo Cleanse, Zero Lather Condition Cleanser & One Condition Ultra Creamy Daily Conditioner	$: L'Oreal EverCurl Hydracharge Shampoo + Conditioner $$: Ouidad PlayCurl Volumizing Shampoo + Conditioner	$: SheaMoisture Curl & Shine Shampoo + Conditioner $$: AG Curl Re:Coil Curl Care Shampoo + Conditioner	$: L'Oreal EverSleek Sulfate-Free Smoothing System™ Intense Smoothing Conditioner $$: Kerastase Nutritive Bain Oleo-Curl Bain Shampoo + Conditioner
kinky	$ OGX Quenching Coconut Curls Shampoo + Conditioner $$ Living Proof Curl Conditioning Wash + Curl Detangling Rinse	$ SheaMoisture Yucca & Plantain Anti-Breakage Strengthening Shampoo + Conditioner $$ Serge Normant Meta Silk Shampoo + Conditioner	$ Nature's Gate Jojoba Revitalizing Shampoo + Conditioner $$ Aveda Be Curly Shampoo + Conditioner	$ Not Your Mother's Kinky Moves Curl Defining Shampoo + Conditioner $$ Carol's Daughter Monoi Repairing Duo

how to traditionally shampoo and condition your red hair

If you have unruly hair, like most redheads do, or if you're simply looking for a controlled look, gorgeous hair starts with this process:

1. First, gently brush your red hair before hopping in the shower. This will keep the locks from tangling when wet and will allow the product to evenly distribute throughout the hair. Use a wide paddle brush with 100% natural boar bristles reinforced with nylon pins. We prefer this type of brush because it's gentler on the hair and never tugs or breaks the ends. It is ideal for all hair lengths and types. The boar bristles evenly distribute the scalp's natural oils to promote shiny, healthy hair.

our "redhead friendly" favorites

$: Conair Mega Ceramic Porcupine Cushion Hair Brush

$$: Denman Medium Grooming Brush Natural Bristle & Nylon Pins

$$$: Mason Pearson Boar Bristle & Nylon Hairbrush

2. After a long day at work or school, who doesn't love a hot shower? Although it is relaxing, your hair hates it! The heat and steam actually deplete the hair of its natural oils and can make it dry and frizzy. Make sure to shower with lukewarm water because it opens up the cuticle, letting your hair know it's time for a wash.

3. Grab your sulfate-free shampoo and squeeze a quarter-size dollop into your hand, rub hands together to lather, then massage evenly over your scalp. If your hair has extra build-up, shampoo twice. This will make sure your hair is fully clean.

4. Next, apply a little under a quarter size of your sulfate-free, paraben-free conditioner, concentrating mainly on the ends. Avoid applying directly to roots to prevent your hair from getting oily. Keep the conditioner on your hair for 2 to 3 minutes to make sure your locks are getting replenished with the product.

Tip #1: When we know we'll be giving our hair a blow out, our favorite shampoo + conditioner set is Kenra Platinum Blow Dry Shampoo and Conditioner.

Tip #2: Brushing your hair with conditioner is okay, BUT the hair should not be soaking wet. If you want to brush in the shower, follow NYC hairstylist, Kiera Doyle's tip on next page.

For curly-haired redheads, brushing curls at any stage can cause them to split and frizz. Squeeze excess water out. Keeping your head far from the running water, apply conditioner from ends through mid-shaft using less and less as you approach the scalp. Work product through with fingers first. Then, using an appropriate brush—either a wide tooth comb or wet brush—use one hand to hold the hair section and the other to brush it. Start at the ends and work your way up. Be gentle. If you feel resistance, stop and comb through from the bottom of the knot up. Do not pull or tug through knots. Wet hair is extra flexible and has the ability to stretch more than it should.

5. Rinse the conditioner out of the hair and blast it with cold water. This will lock in the cuticle, making your hair smooth and shiny!

6. Next, use a microfiber towel, our favorite is by AQUIS. Or, if you're on a budget, simply use a 100% cotton T-shirt. The cotton in the T-shirt is gentler than the fibers in normal towels and will keep your cuticle smooth and noticeably softer. Squeeze the excess moisture out rather than rubbing hair dry, which can cause frizz and breakage. Never brush your hair right after you shower, because it causes breakage. If you have any tangles, gently run your fingers through your hair. Wait until the ends begin to dry before brushing.

We call this six-step method the "RedSHAMPion Process."

alternative cleansers

If you have strong hair strands, curly hair and/or can go a few days without shampooing without any issues, you might enjoy the "no-poo" fad. This term means two things:

1. A cleanser without sulfates. (Get it? There is "no-poo" or harmful chemicals in the product.)

2. The process of using a sulfate-free cleanser *or* no cleanser at all. The process of not using shampoo leads to the most common phrase among hair professionals: co-washing. Co-washing means using a botanical sulfate-free conditioner to wash your hair. You completely skip the shampoo process. By co-washing you're also following the no-poo method.

our "redhead friendly" favorites

$: L'Oreal EverCreme Cleansing Conditioner

$$: UNWASH Bio-Cleansing Conditioner

"A no-shampoo method of cleansing your hair using a product that contains more conditioner than cleanser. Traditionally a 'free-from' product with no harsh ingredients."

—Kiera Doyle, NYC hairstylist

Co-washing is not for everyone, because it purposely skips the shampooing process. Co-washing is not recommended for those with fine or thin hair, because you will need traditional shampoo to keep your locks from appearing thin and lifeless; co-washing conditioners might weigh thin hair down. For redheads with coarse, curly and/or thick hair, you might enjoy co-washing because the conditioning ingredients give hair definition and shine while preventing frizz. If you enjoy the feeling of a thoroughly clean scalp, you might not enjoy this alternative cleanser.

Dry shampoo is another alternative cleanser that gives your red hair the appearance of looking clean since it absorbs the oil that can make hair look dirty. Find the right washing routine that's best for you, whether it's two to three times a week or less, and use dry shampoo every day in between.

our "redhead friendly" favorites

$: Not Your Mother's Clean Freak Dry Shampoo (spray)
$$: Blow Pro Faux Dry Shampoo (powder)

Don't want to break the bank? Cornstarch and baby powder are two great dry shampoo options because they are oil-absorbing. Worried about the residue making your red hair look faded or white? Add a few teaspoons of cinnamon or cocoa powder to the mix. This will turn the product a shade of red. Do not worry! This concoction will not leave your hair looking cake-y. Remember: A little goes a very long way. Depending on your hair length, apply a quarter size amount to the scalp, especially where it is most oily. It will quickly absorb into the hair strands.

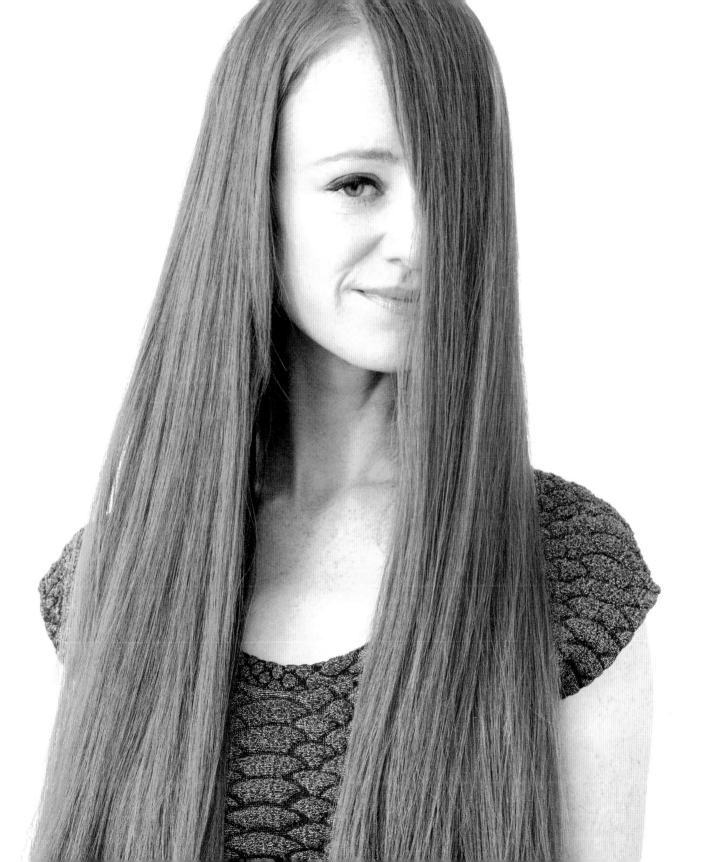

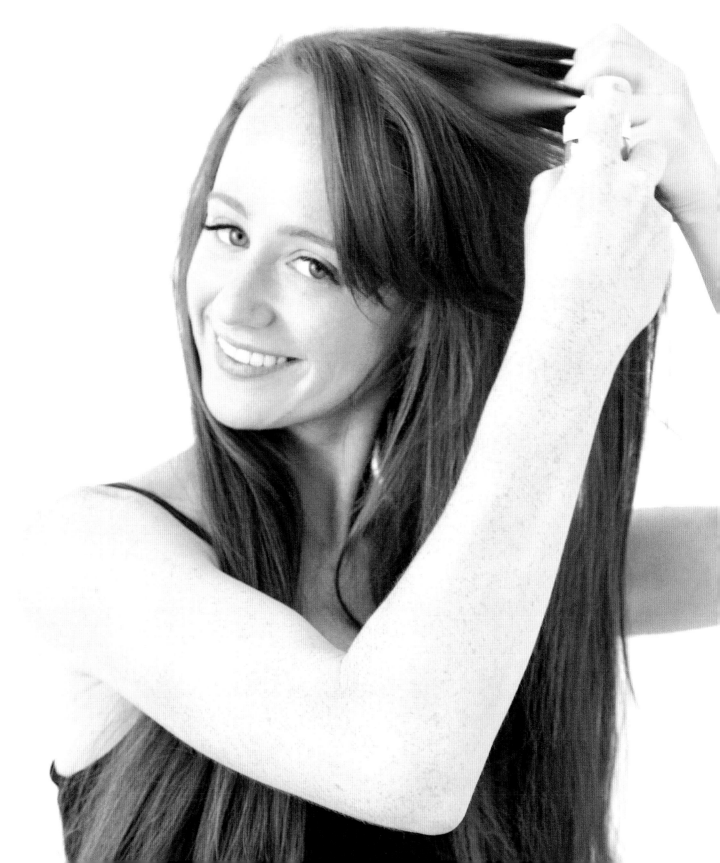

how to use dry shampoo

Whether you decide to use a professional dry shampoo or a DIY product, simply place a quarter-size amount in your palm and apply to the places where the hair looks oily. If you have a mane of red hair, like most redheads do, divide your hair into sections and apply the dry shampoo into each section. To avoid any white residue showing, use your fingers to rub the dry shampoo into your roots. After application, we like to use a brush to even out the product. It is optional, but we prefer to use a hair straightener to set and style the look. If you love your curly or wavy locks, you can use a curling iron too.

Adrienne only washes her hair once every seven days! The natural oils keep her hair strong and healthy. On the fourth or fifth day, she uses a dry shampoo to keep her hair looking fresh, and by the sixth or seventh day, her hair is in a ponytail or ballerina bun.

the best hair styling tools for your red hair

Let's admit it, redheads never *really* have bad hair days. The hair color is so beautiful, how can it ever look anything but stunning? But styling tools can make a look go from pretty to drop-dead gorgeous in seconds.

1

blow-dryer

Invest in a good hair dryer because it will make your hair smoother and shinier and cuts your time when drying it. We suggest a ceramic dryer as they emit non–damaging heat and distribute heat evenly across your head. Result: Silky, non–frizzy red hair.

"redhead friendly" tip: Make sure to clean out the air vent located at the end of your blow dryer. This will prolong the life of your dryer and eliminate overheating.

our "redhead friendly" favorites

$: Conair Ionic Ceramic Cord-Keeper Hair Dryer

$$: SuperSolano The Original

Should you flip your hair over when you're blow-drying? If you want volume, this is how to do it. But it's very important to point the blow-dryer in the direction of the hair cuticle or else your hair will turn into a big, frizzy mess! If you blow-dry from the root to end, you'll always have shiny results.

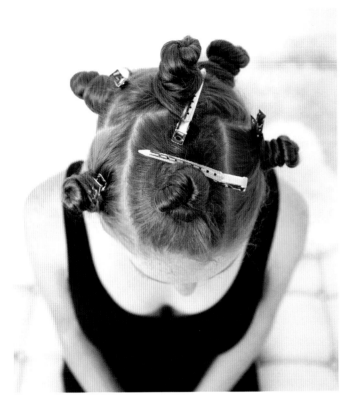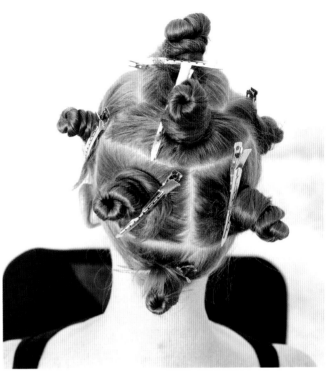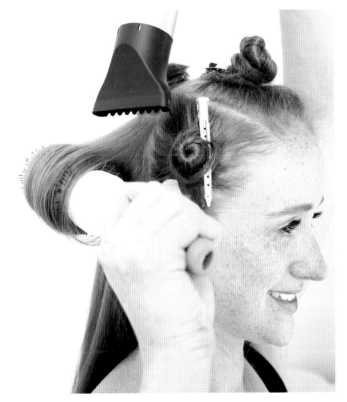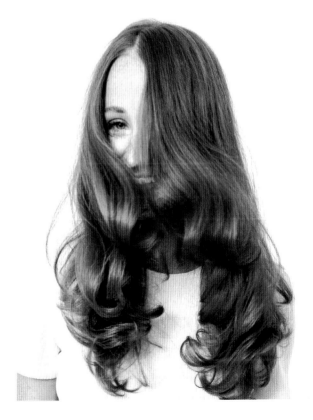

curling iron

½ inch (13 mm), ¾ inch (19 mm), 1 inch (2.5 cm)…oh my! The size of your curling iron barrel depends on how big you want your curls. We suggest 1 inch (2.5 cm) or more for longer, thicker red hair, and ½ inch (13 mm) to ¾ inch (19 mm) for shorter hair. This will give your red locks the capability to create bouncy, big curls. Curling irons do not have to be pricey. Opt for one that has adjustable heat settings.

our "redhead friendly" favorite

$: Hot Tools Gold Curling Iron

It may be bit challenging to figure out the clamp on a curling iron. That's why we love a wand. It's a clamp-less iron that gives you the ability to easily create curls. Simply wrap each section of your hair onto the wand from root to end, always making sure to curl outward with the opposite hand. Left-sided curls are done by holding the wand with the right hand and wrapping the curls with the left hand, while right-sided curls are done by holding the wand with left hand and wrapping the curls with the right hand. Hold for a few seconds and release.

our "redhead friendly" favorites

$: Bed Head Curlipops Textured Curling Wand Iron

$$: Sedu Revolution Clipless Curling Iron

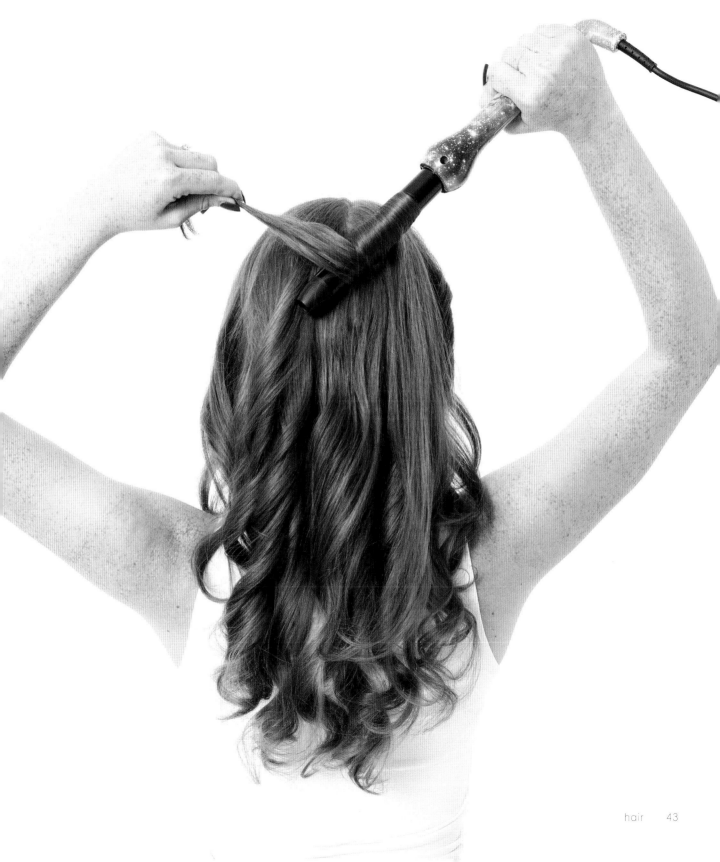

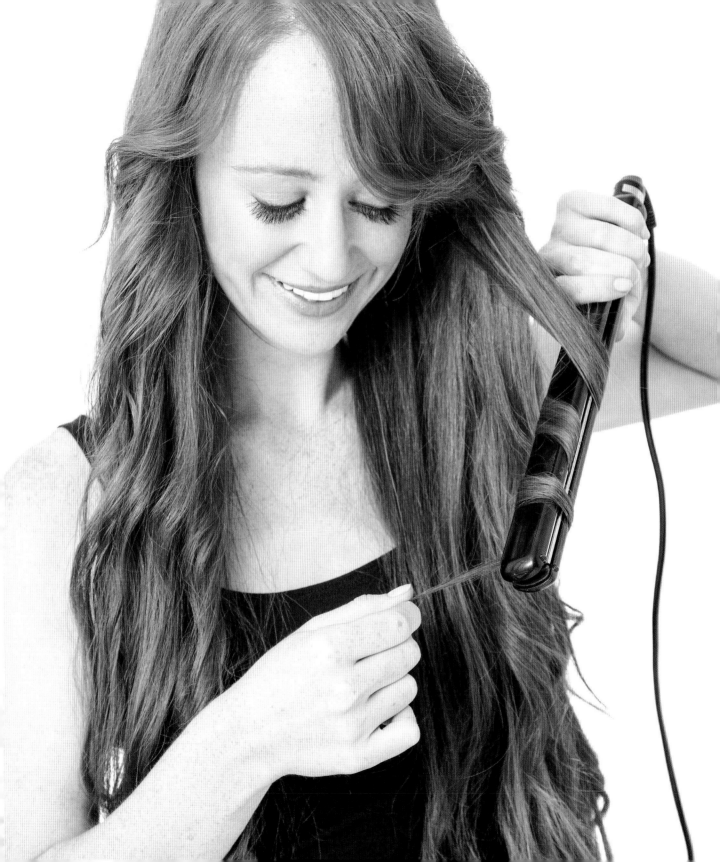

"redhead friendly" tip

You can use your straightening iron as a curling iron! Here's how:

1. Make sure the straightening iron is on and well heated.

2. Separate hair into sections. When curling on the left side, use iron in the right hand. When curling on the right side, use iron in the left hand. Always making sure your hand is away from you when creating the curls.

3. Take a small piece of one of the hair sections. If your sections are too big, you won't get desired curls. The smaller the sections, the tighter the curl.

4. Wrap the middle of each small section of hair around the iron and pull down, constantly moving in 180-degree movements and keeping the iron outward with your elbow lifted. The position of the straightening iron and elbow is key to a flawless curl.

5. During this quick movement, never release the straightening iron or else you will get dents in your hair instead of curls.

get Ariel's, from Disney's *The Little Mermaid*, look:

Step 1: Wrap dry, clean hair around 1 inch (2.5 cm) curling iron or wand to create varied, unstructured waves throughout hair.

Step 2: Finish with a firm hairspray to make sure the hair stays in place.

hot rollers

Not a fan of curling irons? Or do you simply not have the time? Electric hot rollers are a great way to easily add curls throughout your hair. They typically come in heat-protectant setting cases. Some sets come with a multitude of different sizes, ranging from ¾ inch (19 mm) to 2 inches (5 cm) wide. The smaller the roller, the smaller and tighter the curl; the bigger the roller, the more voluminous and bigger the curls. Simply plug in the case and wait five minutes for the rollers to heat up before using.

We love to put in hot rollers right at the very beginning of our "getting ready" routine. That way, once our makeup is done and outfit is chosen, our curls are done and ready for the world to see.

"redhead friendly" tip: For those with naturally frizzy, coarse hair, it is always suggested that your hair is blown out straight before using hot rollers. That way, the curls look bouncy and beautiful. You never want to go from a wild mane to rollers. Take the time to make your hair silky prior to using rollers.

Self-Holding Velcro Rollers: These are perfect if you are traveling, because they do not take up much room and still give great results. Choose velcro rollers that do not require pins or clips, because they're much easier! Make sure to take small sections of hair and use the 'Hot Rollers' directions above. Use a bit of heat protectant and wrap the hair around the rollers, then apply blow-dryer heat to the head to lock in the curls. Keep in for 30 to 45 minutes—the longer, the better.

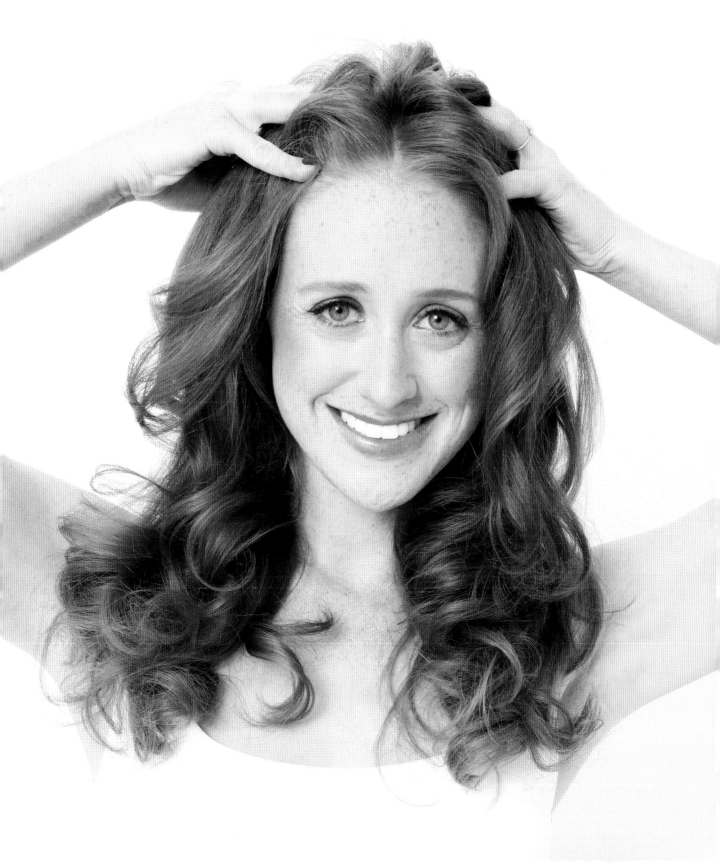

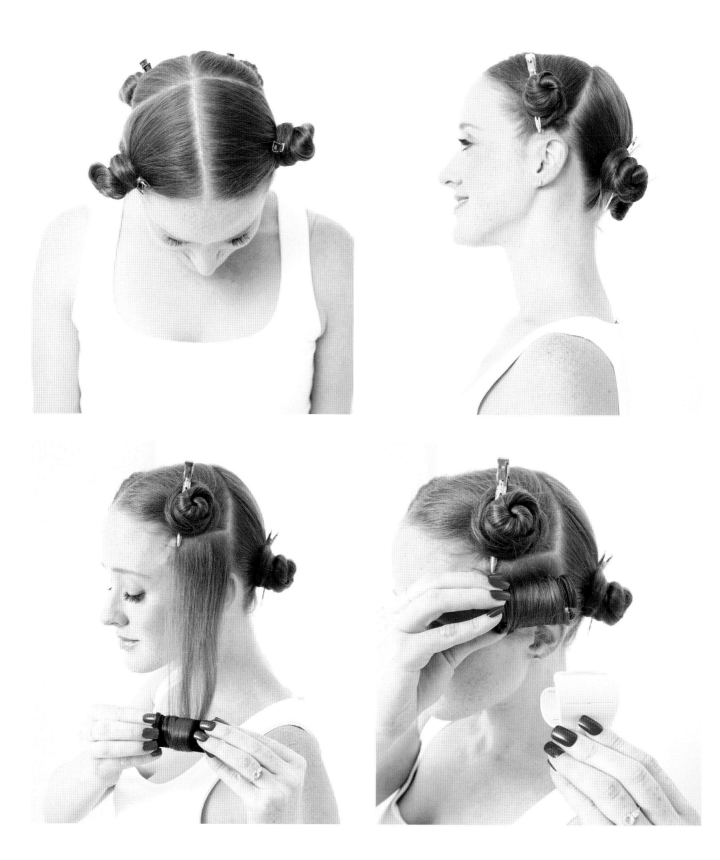

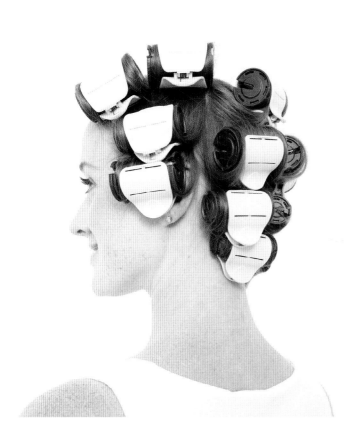
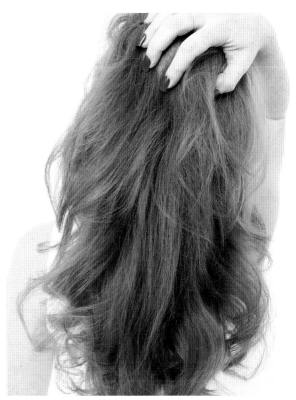

How to Use: Lightly apply a heat protectant serum to the ends of your hair to prevent the rollers from damaging it. Section off hair into fourths, then section off each fourth into smaller sections so you aren't wrapping too much hair around each roller. Next take your roller and place in the middle of your section and take the end of each hair strand and wrap it around the roller. Once you get to the middle, roll it to your head. To make sure the rollers stay in place, secure each roller with a clip. Let set for 20 to 30 minutes. The longer you have them in, the more defined the curls will be and the longer they'll last. When ready, gently take each roller out one by one. Do not yank or pull them out as you do not want breakage to occur. Once the rollers are out, run your fingers through the hair and spray hairspray throughout to lock it all in.

our "redhead friendly" favorite

BaByliss Pro Nano Titanium Ionic Roller Set

flat iron

Commonly known as a hair straightener. We have had a flat iron in our bathroom since we were teenagers. It was a must-have then and it is certainly a must-have now. Purchase a high-quality, ceramic hair iron. It will cause less damage to your red hair, while leaving it smooth and full of shine.

What is the best temperature to straighten hair? What's too hot? Kiera Doyle breaks it down for us: "Most flat irons go up to 450°F (232°C) but that's usually not necessary unless hair is extremely resistant. If you have to use high heat, make sure to use heat protectors and keep the flat iron moving. Comb hair thoroughly before running the hot iron over each section, this will help the flat iron glide more easily over the hair and not get tangled."

"redhead friendly" tips

+ Embrace your natural hair texture. Only opt for a hair iron if you want a sleek, straight look.

+ Mini flat irons are a great choice if you're traveling or have very short hair. Our favorite: BaByliss PRO Nano Titanium Mini Straightening Iron in ½ inch (13 mm).

recommended temperatures

Fine or fragile hair: 250°F (121°C) or lower

Thick or coarse hair: 300°F (149°C) or higher

our "redhead friendly" favorites

$: Hot Tools Digital Salon Flat Iron w/ Titanium Plates

$$: Chi Ultra CHI Red Ceramic Flat Iron

diffuser

Do you have naturally frizzy, curly red hair? A diffuser is for you. Many blow-dryers come with a diffuser attachment and they are super easy to use.

How to Use: Starting at your roots, slowly work the fingers of the diffuser in a circular motion on a low heat setting. Don't stay on a section for too long, as you don't want to damage your red locks. The result: natural, effortless curls.

Note: When purchasing a blow-dryer, make sure it comes with a diffuser nozzle. This will eliminate finding a diffuser attachment to fit your dryer.

Get Merida from Disney's *Brave* Look: Separate damp hair like you're going to make pigtails, squeeze styling product onto your palms, then apply it on one side of the hair first. Start to scrunch up your hair with your hands. Do the same routine on the other side. Use a diffuser to diffuse your hair and create the curl quicker. It will also give volume to the hair without frizz. Use hairspray to maintain the curls.

Look for these properties on a styling-product bottle:

+ Heat protection
+ Styling protectant

+ Anti-breakage
+ Thermal protectant

It is always suggested to use a dime- to nickel-size amount of product throughout the hair, then use your desired tool. It's important that you do not apply too much or you could do the opposite of what the product is supposed to do. If product is sprayed or applied too intensely on a section, the styling tool could almost cook the hair and cause it to break off.

If you're a redhead who uses heat-styling tools such as blow-dryers, curling irons and flat irons, it's important to choose styling products that contain heat-protectant properties to keep the hair safe.

hair brushes

We get very overwhelmed in the hairbrush aisle. There are too many to choose from! Here's a quick 101 on which ones are great for redheads:

tail comb

Great for creating parts and smoothing out any hair strands once styled.

Our Favorite: Ace Combs Tail Comb for fine to medium hair.

wide comb

Use a wide comb on damp hair to untangle red strands.

Our Favorite: Cricket Ultra Smooth Conditioning Comb infused with argan oil and olive oil.

paddle brush

Usually large and wide. Great for long, wavy or straight locks.

Our Favorite: Conair Mega Ceramic Porcupine Cushion Hair Brush

4

vent brush

Great for a redhead with short hair and looking to spend a small amount of time blow-drying.

Our favorite: Revlon Tunnel Vent Brush

teasing brush

Use when you're looking to tease strands and add overall volume to hair.

Our Favorite: Cricket Amped Up Teasing Brush

6

round brush

Use when blow-drying hair. Great for creating bounce. For longer hair, use a larger hair barrel. For shorter hair, use a shorter hair barrel.

Our Favorite: Chi Turbo Round Brush

different bristles on a round brush

+ Boar Bristle: Great for regular to coarse hair.

+ Nylon & Boar: Great for fine hair.

+ Synthetic (Ceramic, Ion): Great for regular to medium hair.

"redhead friendly" tip: Always look at the bristles. If they are close together, then they are perfect for fine hair.

our "redhead friendly" favorite hairbrush brands

Spornette Porcupine & Mason Pearson

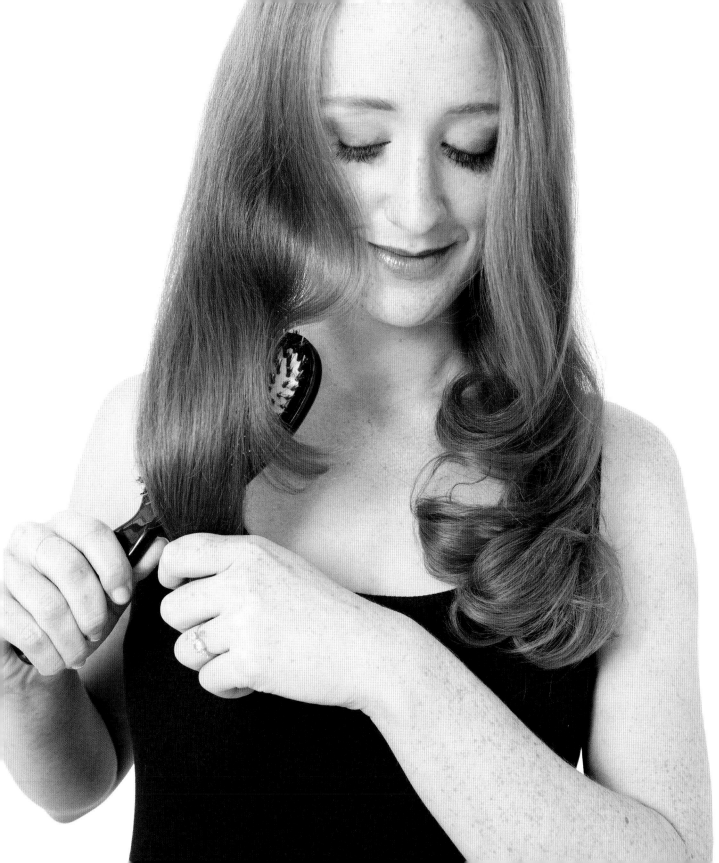

how to brush red hair

Whether wet or dry, you should always brush red hair from its ends to roots. Hair strands are fragile and this will eliminate any breakage. Avoid brushing wet hair because the hair cuticle is vulnerable. Wait until it is at least 70 percent dry.

Since redheads have thicker hair than any other color, you might notice increased shedding when brushing or shampooing. It's normal to shed between 50 and 100 red hairs a day.

"How can I miss you when I find your hair everywhere?"

"redhead friendly" tips

+ Use a silk pillowcase to keep red hair silky and less frizzy. The silk allows the hair to move at night, while cotton pillowcases create friction, which can lead to breakage and dryness.

+ Should you or should you not brush your hair before bed? If the hair is fine, you can because the texture allows brushes to soften the strands. "If you have curly hair, definitely do not brush hair before bed," says NYC hairstylist Kiera Doyle. "If the goal is to wake up with smooth locks, part hair in a natural part all the way down the nape of the neck, twist hair into two low buns and pin with redhead bobby pins."

take care of hair brushes

Wash brushes in warm water with a bit of shampoo (baby shampoo works, too), rinse and let brushes dry on a towel overnight.

hair accessories for styling
redhead bobby pins and hair ties

When we were getting ready for prom season in high school, we realized that there weren't bobby pins or hair ties for redheads. We were forced to use blonde, brunette and black pins and ties. Once we launched our website, we made the decision to begin creating the first hair accessories for redheads.

There are many different types of red hair. The three most common are copper, classic red and deep auburn. We created a bobby pin for each of those redheads and put them all in one easy package. Then, we created hair ties in these three shades, as well as other variations. The accessories camouflage into the hair of some redheads, but the bobby pins have been primarily designed to make red hair pop.

tips for wearing redhead bobby pins

Wavy Side Down: Despite what everyone else thinks, bobby pins are meant to be worn wavy side down. The wavy side, aka the grips, are designed to hold hair in place.

Make Those Redhead Bobby Pins Sticky: By spraying pins with hairspray, they will be able to hold hair all day. Place your bobby pins on a napkin and spray for 1 to 2 seconds with a strong-hold hairspray. Dry shampoo will work well too.

our "redhead friendly" favorite

Salon Care Croco Clip

Don't forget crocodile styling clips! These funky clamps are great
for separating and securing hair into sections. But don't use clips directly on
styled hair, or else dents will form. If you need hair (mainly bangs) to be held off your
face, place a square piece of paper towel on the hair, then apply clip
on top of the paper towel to prevent denting.

"redhead friendly" styling products

Our mother has board straight hair and did not know how to combat our red manes. So she did what most moms in those days did: cut our hair into short bobs. Of course, our hair then grew outward and the frizz multiplied.

We'll never forget the day in middle school when we discovered hair tools, specifically straightening irons and anti-frizz styling creme. We said to each other with excitement, "Can you believe these exist?" From then on, we were hooked. And it didn't stop there. We tested serums, oils, mousses, gels, hairsprays and more.

"I find it empowering to style a redhead celebrity because the hair color helps the look to stand out, and being a part of that feels timeless and iconic."

—Marcus Francis, celebrity hair stylist

hairspray

Ideal for all hair types. Every redhead (natural or "by choice") should own a bottle of hairspray that holds hair in place and adds texture and volume. It never fails and always has your back when maintaining a certain look.

Strong-hold hairsprays are great for hairstyles that require long-lasting holds. Medium-hold hairsprays are great for everyday hairstyles that require a light mist and not much hold, such as a blowout.

How to: Spray in constant motion (left to right) at least 12 inches (30 cm) from your red hair. Spraying too close to the hair will create product buildup.

"redhead friendly" tip: Spray a little hairspray on a toothbrush or your fingertips to tame any baby red hairs, especially after using a straightening iron.

our "redhead friendly" favorites

$: Medium Hold: Kenra Professional Perfect Medium Spray 13

$$: Strong Hold: Elnett Satin Hairspray Strong Hold

hair gel

Ideal for medium to coarse hair. Calling all you curly haired redheads! Hair gel got a bad rap with the 80s *the-bigger-the-hair-the-better* trend. But hair gel is making a comeback. It's great for curly locks, and when used properly can really define and structure each strand. Use it on wavy hair to add dimension or apply to curls to minimize frizz.

How To: Apply gel to damp hair from the ends, working your way up to the roots. Scrunch the hair as you apply the product. This will add extra volume and give definition to each curl.

"redhead friendly" tip: Make sure you're using the right hair gel or else you will be stuck with a crunchy, greasy red mess.

our favorite "redhead friendly" hair gels

$: Matrix Style Link Super Fixer Strong Hold Gel

$$: Davines This Is A Medium Hold Modeling Gel

mousse

Ideal for fine to medium hair. An oldie but goodie for a good reason! Hair mousse is great for adding soft, weightless hold while adding volume, texture and dimension.

How To: Make sure to shake the bottle before using because the ingredients that make up mousse separate. If you don't do this, the mousse will come out watery. Put a golf-ball-size amount in the palm of your hand, rub together with both hands (or else it will liquefy) and apply from the ends to the root so your hair doesn't look weighed down.

"redhead friendly" tip: Mousse is great for those with thin or fine hair because it gives the illusion of volume and texture. For ultimate volume, divide hair into sections or flip head over and apply mousse throughout hair before blow-drying. This will give the hair more dimension because the roots of the hair are actually being lifted.

our "redhead friendly" favorites

$: TRESemmé Flawless Curls Extra Hold Mousse

$$: Oribe Surfcomber Tousled Texture Mousse

styling creme

Ideal for all hair types. It's all about control, and styling creme knows how to do it. It eliminates frizz and preps hair before styling. Even though it is neither a gel nor mousse, it works like both.

How To: Apply a quarter-size amount onto palms, rub together and apply to damp hair. The product holds the hair in place with light hold until it dries.

"redhead friendly" tips

+ Use styling creme as a deep conditioner by applying it to ends of hair, securing into a bun and rinsing out the next morning.

+ If you have curly hair, after the creme dries in the hair, lightly comb the hair for gorgeous, frizz-free curls.

our "redhead friendly" favorites

$: Paul Mitchell Express Style Quick Slip Styling Cream

$$: WEN by Chaz Dean Sweet Almond Mint Anti-Frizz Styling Creme

sea salt spray

Natural-looking beach hair to the rescue! Easily attain a beach look with salt sprays and keep locks hydrated and mermaid–like. But beware! Many salt sprays actually dry out the hair in the process.

How To: Spray throughout damp hair and scrunch. Avoid the roots because you don't want the product concentrated on the scalp; instead focus on the bottom and mid-shaft where you want to see the waves form.

"redhead friendly" tip: Take it with you to the beach and apply on damp, ocean-soaked hair. Or for a more soft, subtle wave, do as NYC hairstylist Kiera Doyle does and rub a few drops of oil/smoothing cream into your hands and run through your hair after the sea salt spray is applied.

our "redhead friendly" favorites

$: Not Your Mother's Beach Babe Texturizing Sea Salt Spray

$$: Bumble and Bumble Sea Salt Spray

hair oil

Ideal for medium to thick hair. Hair oils are oil-based products that provide shine and act as great deep conditioners.

How To: Apply a dime-size amount onto palms, rub together and apply to damp hair. Only use on the ends or else you will experience a greasy, oily scalp.

"redhead friendly" tip: Argan oil is a great oil option. It gives hair a silky and lustrous finish. It does not weigh down hair, accumulate residue or make hair look greasy and unwashed.

our "redhead friendly" favorites

$: Moroccanoil Pure Argan Oil

$$: UNITE U Argan Oil

"I recommend hair oils if the hair has a coarse texture to it, which then it will cut down on styling by helping to smooth the hair cuticle. If the hair is on the finer side, I wouldn't use oils as they tend to make the hair greasy and weigh it down."

—Marcus Francis, celebrity hair stylist

styling powder

Ideal for all hair types. Styling powder is intended for teasing and adding *vol-vol-vol-volume!* It comes as a white powder and can often be mistaken for dry shampoo.

How To: Apply the powder directly to dry roots. Rub into red hair as much as possible.

"redhead friendly" tip: Add volume to a specific hair section by teasing it. Simply section the top of the head and add a few dashes of powder to the scalp. Rub into the roots and gently brush downward with a tail comb or teasing brush comb. Make sure to tease in fast, rhythmic motions. Repeat until you have achieved your desired volume. Gently brush the teased hair to secure and volumize. Remember: the bigger the tease, the bigger the red hair.

our "redhead friendly" favorites

$: Rock Your Hair Bombshell Big Hair Powder

$$: Kenra Professional Platinum Texture Powder 4

pomade

Ideal for short red hair. This product is best described as a greasy or waxy substance that is used to style hair. It's a great option for a redhead with short hair because it doesn't weigh hair down, and you have complete control over how much you apply and where you apply it.

How To: Start off by applying a dime-size amount of product to the index and middle fingers and rub together. Apply pomade directly onto hair strands, dry or wet. This product is very buildable, so start with a little and work your way up.

"redhead friendly" tip: Creating a sleek hairstyle? After styling, apply a penny-size amount of pomade to ends and any flyaways.

our "redhead friendly" favorites

$: got2B Defiant Define + Shine Pomade

$$: TIGI Bed Head Manipulator

the five commandments for prepping & styling red hair

①

Thou shalt not use products with sulfates or parabens.

②

Thou shalt not use a towel to dry hair.

③

Thou shalt not use extra-hot water when washing hair.

④

Thou shalt not use an inexpensive brush. Invest in quality to keep red hair looking great.

⑤

Thou shalt LOVE thy red hair!

SPF for your red hair

It is always recommended to use a hat, scarf or head accessory to keep hair safe from the harmful effects of the sun. But it's also equally important to use an SPF spray for your hair. Yes, they do exist! It protects red hair and scalp from damaging rays and keeps hair (both natural and "by choice") from fading. Let's admit it: sunburn on the scalp is the worst! It burns and flakes after a few days, making it look like you have loads of dandruff. To prevent this from happening, invest in an SPF spray for the hair and scalp.

How To: Simply spray evenly throughout dry or wet hair. For maximum results, it is best to use the product when the hair is dry because it will penetrate through hair strands faster and give the scalp more coverage.

our "redhead friendly" favorites

$: Aveda Sun Care Protective Hair Veil

$$: Shiseido Refreshing Sun Protection Spray

If the scalp does get sunburned, perform the following steps:

1. Wash hair and apply aloe vera juice directly to the scalp. Aloe vera can be found at your local health food store. Let it soak into the scalp overnight and rinse with cold (never hot!) water.

2. Another easy at-home remedy is to apply organic Dijon mustard to the burn, keeping it on until you feel the scalp beginning to cool. Gently shampoo and condition hair. After drying it, apply coconut oil to the burn, letting it soak into scalp overnight. Rinse with cold water.

our "redhead friendly" favorite

$: Spectrum Organic Coconut Oil

natural redheads

if you're thinking of dyeing your hair or are battling fading locks:

"Red is the rarest and most unique hair color. You were genetically chosen to be special, you are lucky, so do not be afraid to wear your red hair with pride. I had one client who had a beautiful shade of red that she did not like, and would ask to get a lot of very light pale blonde to cover up her natural light strawberry ginger hair color. It did not complement her well and I convinced her to gloss over the highlights to a lighter copper color. Two weeks later, she met her future husband who approached her in a bar and complimented her on her gorgeous natural red hair!"

—James Corbett, Clairol color director, celebrity colorist, beauty expert and proud uncle to natural redheads

stephanie's story

Growing up, I always felt out of place because of my red hair. I wanted to hide every strand of red, whether it was with a hat, a headband or what I later turned to, bleach. My mother, who thought I needed to get this I-hate-my-hair phase out of my system, gave me permission to get highlights when I was in the sixth grade. I didn't stop there. I continued to color my hair for the next seven years. After years of coloring, the highlights soon spread into thick strands of blonde, and before I knew it, I was a full-blown blonde, platinum to the max. As soon as my red would show through, I would make an appointment to get a retouch of bleach right at the root. I did not want a trace of red to show.

I remember running my hands through my hair and it felt rubbery and dead. The years of dyeing my hair had damaged it so badly that even the best leave-in conditioners could not help my once beautiful curly red strands.

After years of scheduling hair appointments, dishing out hundreds of dollars and sitting in the salon chair for hours, I decided to stop the bleaching during my sophomore year of college and do the one thing I should have done years back: embrace my natural hues.

I remember that exact moment I made the commitment to let my red hair grow, and I still get chills thinking about it. I was going back to my roots (no pun intended), and it was about time! The days of hiding my inner and outer redhead were over.

I was finally Stephanie, the redhead. I was and *still* am proud of it.

Because natural red hair holds its pigment more than other colors,
it is harder to dye. This might be the hair gods' way of making it difficult for
natural redheads to dye their hair!

natural redheads

if you're thinking of dyeing your hair, read the five reasons
why stephanie wishes she hadn't

(1)

I spent years blending in with the crowd, when I was born to stand out.

(2)

Countless hours and money (over $4,000) were spent that I will never get back.

(3)

I regret not being referred to as a redhead for the seven years everyone
called me a blonde. I feel as if my friends and family, during those blonde years,
really did not know or see the real me.

(4)

My hair looked like straw because it was so dead. It took about three years
for my healthy hair to grow back.

(5)

To mask the appearance of being a redhead, I purchased expensive makeup products
to cover my freckles. Years later, I hardly wear makeup and my freckles are my true
accessory. I feel incredibly free, and most important, I feel like ME!

how to keep red hair from fading

maintenance tips for natural or "by choice" redheads

"Shop for a colorist like you would shop for a dress. As a natural redhead, I never thought the day would come when I would go gray. Now, the only problem is making my hair look the same red as it was naturally. A redhead must have a great colorist to match their natural hair. You can't go to *anyone*; it has to be someone good. My advice is to take a picture NOW of your red hair, or find a photo you love, and when the time comes, you can tell your hairdresser, 'This is the color I want.'"

—Felicia Milewicz, ex-beauty director of *Glamour* magazine for 40 years

Looking to enhance red hair? Want to preserve and illuminate colored strands? Color-depositing shampoos and conditioners naturally deposit color in the hair as you wash it. If you're a natural redhead, add this to your beauty routine a few times a week, and if you're a redhead "by choice," use this regularly to lengthen time in-between trips to the salon.

our "redhead friendly" favorites

$$: Davines Alchemic Red

$$$: Pureology Reviving Red

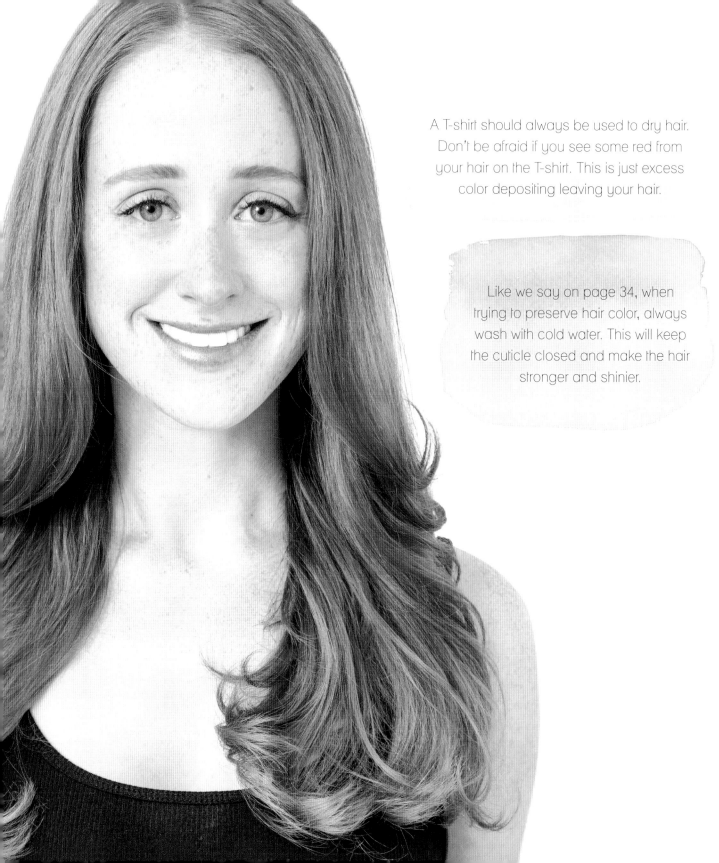

A T-shirt should always be used to dry hair. Don't be afraid if you see some red from your hair on the T-shirt. This is just excess color depositing leaving your hair.

Like we say on page 34, when trying to preserve hair color, always wash with cold water. This will keep the cuticle closed and make the hair stronger and shinier.

hair gloss treatment

"For a redhead to color her hair, it can be a scary process! I always approach a natural redhead going through browning out or dulling of a once beautiful natural red with a conservative approach."

—Rona O'Connor, Lukaro Salon & Spa owner and celebrity colorist

Glosses are a great way to add a deep conditioner to hair, while enhancing its natural red tones. They can be done either at home or at a professional hair salon. Regardless make sure to stick to a semi-permanent gloss. It'll boost the hair for 6 to 8 weeks, naturally washing away so you won't see any drastic changes after a few weeks.

Stephanie loves getting glosses, especially during the fall and winter months when she wants to enhance her red and add a deep tone to the strands. Glosses are great for someone who is looking for minimal maintenance and just wants a little pop of color to enhance her natural hue.

Another name for hair gloss is demi-permanent.

our "redhead friendly" favorite

$: Clairol Natural Instincts Shine Happy

"Ask the colorist to enhance your red hues with a demi-permanent or gloss as a first line of defense. Most redheads lose their vibrancy and 'get dusty' before they actually go gray. Demi-permanents help boost your color without heavy commitment. Anyone is a great candidate for a hair gloss. They can be a great way to add a touch of vibrancy and give your strands a much needed boost of color. Glosses can be used alone or in conjunction with an at-home root application to refresh the color on the midshaft and ends of the hair. Or they can be used alone for a subtle boost and enhancement."

—James Corbett, Clairol color director, celebrity colorist, beauty expert and proud uncle to natural redheads

hair glaze

Add shine and smoothness to red locks with clear glazes. This can be done at home or in a salon.

our "redhead friendly" favorite

$: John Frieda Clear Shine Luminous Hair Glaze

henna

Henna is a reddish dye obtained from powdered leaves of the *Lawsonia inermis* plant, used as a cosmetic and industrial dye. It is a great option if the hair is fading or you're looking for a little boost. Henna can be reapplied as frequently as needed without damage because it is a great hair conditioner, which will soften and add shine to the hair. Unlike hair colors and dyes, henna is totally safe for use and can be used as many times as needed.

You must avoid henna if you have had or currently receive chemical hair treatments.

tips to help you achieve red hair
using henna

1. Make sure to buy pure henna with no other ingredients in it. Body-art henna that can be applied on the hands, also known as *mehndi*, is the best henna to buy.

2. Use 100 to 500 grams of good-quality henna, depending on the length of your hair. Mix with warm water to make a smooth paste.

3. Cover the bowl and leave it in a dark place at room temperature for at least 12 hours. It is preferable to wash and dry hair before applying henna.

4. Apply cream or petroleum jelly the hairline, forehead and ears to prevent the henna from staining the skin. Put on protective gloves, as henna stains everything it touches.

5. Divide the hair in half and cover every strand with the henna paste to get an even coverage. Henna can be quite thick, making it difficult to apply if you have long, coarse hair. If you find it difficult to apply it yourself, then have someone apply it for you.

6. When the entire head is covered, place a plastic cap over the hair to prevent it from drying out. Henna doesn't work if it dries out. Leave it on for 3 to 4 hours.

7. When it is time to rinse the henna out, wash the hair with tap water and do not use shampoo. Hair might appear super bright red the first day while it's undergoing oxidation. Gradually, the color will deepen. Avoid using hot styling tools right away, as they will dry out the hair.

how to take the red plunge

"Working on red hair has been my favorite, as a more challenging color, since the beginning of my career. I love being able to add multiple hues, like a natural redheaded child would have. I love seeing the reflection of golds, coppers and even ruby undertones. It's always a fun color to create since there are so many variations. I like to think of it as a painter's color. Red is expressive, happy and uplifting."

—Rona O'Connor, Lukaro Salon & Spa owner and celebrity colorist

at home

"For going red at home, I would suggest first trying a red color tone that is closest to your natural level/shade."

—Chelsey Pickthorn, owner of Pickthorn Salon in Brooklyn
and a Davines educated colorist

Professionals will always recommend that redheads never darken or lighten their hair permanently at home. Opt for a rinse or gloss because it washes out in ten to fourteen washes and the color is natural looking. Never overlap new color with old color, or else you will have different shades and a build up of color.

at the salon

"A good consultation is key before you begin. Specify the color of red you are trying to achieve. Do you want to be a redhead that whispers, talks or shouts? Communicate if you are looking to be a more natural looking redhead or if you want to be bolder.

Pictures are a great way to show your colorist what you are looking for because one person's idea of red is not the same as another's. You would be surprised how many women in my salon think they have red hair, or that their hair looks reddish, when it just has some warmth to their brown or blonde shade! It is okay to bring two sets of pictures, one set being what you want and the other demonstrating what you do not want."

—James Corbett, Clairol color director, celebrity colorist, beauty expert and proud uncle to natural redheads

what color red is right for you?

"When choosing the right hair tone, there are a few other
things you want to take into consideration, like skin tone.
But you can tell a lot by eye color."

—Kiera Doyle, NYC hairstylist

For warm-colored eyes: *Green, golden brown or light hazel.* Warm reds such as
copper-reds will usually be a very good fit.

For cool-colored eyes: *Blue or gray.* Cooler reds like red-red, red-violets and burgundy
are recommended.

For black eyes: "This is a blank slate," Doyle says. "I would use skin tone to determine
the right shade. Usually they are neutral and can choose many different reds."

For brown eyes: Browns can be warm or cool, but it's important to look at the skin. If
they're neutral, they can rock any tone.

Always consult with your hairstylist to see which color is perfect for you.

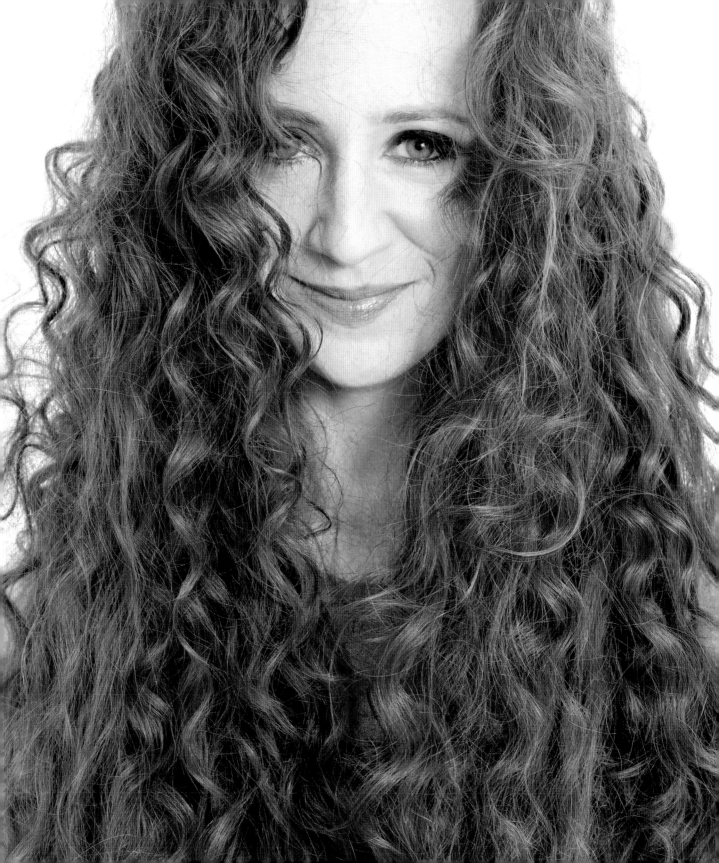

embracing the mane

"You're never going to look boring. Everybody will remember you."

—Julie Klausner, Duchess of Comedy

Grace Coddington, *Vogue's* quirky, outspoken creative director, has the most beautiful red hair. Her hair cannot be tamed, and it has become her signature look. Throughout the years, she has inspired us to embrace our natural, sometimes frizzy and always out of control locks. Women cannot deny that certain hairstyles make them feel a certain way, and although our hair is always stereotyped as being connected with a "crazy" personality, we've discovered when we rock our manes, we feel a fire inside of us, and our feisty personalities are loud and proud.

Do not feel pressured to straighten or change your hair. *Don't tame it! Let it set you free!*

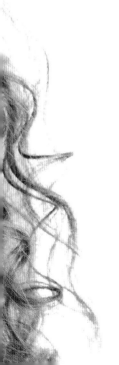

how to go from frizzy to silky

If you read the above and agree but still want silky hair from time to time, the good news is it's easy to accomplish.

For steps 1 to 6, use the RedSHAMPion Process (pages 32–34).

7. Apply a heat-protectant product to the hair to keep red hair protected throughout the styling process.

8. Using crocodile hair clips, divide hair into manageable sections. Section off the top, sides and bottoms.

9. Use a round brush (page 53) and begin blow-drying hair. The shape of the brush allows you to wrap the hair around to add extra bounce.

10. Use a ceramic hair dryer with a nozzle attached (page 40) and make sure the nozzle is always pointing downward. Take the brush and secure it underneath the section at the hairline.

11. The other thing that needs to change is the setting on the blow-dryer. High heat and high air may seem like the best choice, but unless you're a professional, using that combination can leave you with a frizzy mess. Around the hairline, where the hair is most sensitive, turn the setting down to medium (or low, if you have curly hair), and rely on the tension you're creating to smooth out the hair. Once you complete a section, wrap the hair one last time with the round brush and give it a cool blast (like you do in the shower) to help hold its shape and prevent frizz.

"redhead friendly" tip: Hot air shapes hair, cool air sets the shape. Many redheads skip this step, which is why some results do not last.

12. Using the heat of the blow-dryer and the round brush, begin pulling the brush down the hair, then back up in quick movements. Closely apply heat while you perform this step and continue to wrap hair around the brush. Repeat this process until the hair is dry.

13. If you still think the hair is frizzy, use a straightening iron and straighten each piece, section by section. The straightener will flatten the hair strands, giving hair a silky, frizz-free look.

14. Always complete styles with a styling product (page 57) to add shine and protect the hair from harmful outdoor elements. We always prefer a dime-size squirt of hair serum and a quick spritz of hairspray to lock it all in.

Putting your hair in a bun or side braid is another fun option if you're crunched for time. Stephanie loves wrapping her hair in a low bun and securing it with a redhead bobby pin (a hair clip creates a dent at the ends) for a few hours.

Another great tip is dividing your hair into two low ponytails (aka pigtails) and wrapping them individually. Wrap the right pigtail counterclockwise and secure with a pin. Wrap the left pigtail clockwise and secure with a pin. This will make sure curls are going in different directions, making for more movement and overall bounce once you take hair down. Keep in hair for 1 to 2 hours.

Adrienne gets weekly blowouts. Since she puts her hair in the hands of experts, she notices her hair is longer, stronger and healthier. Discover a local blow-dry bar and treat yourself!

how to combat hair issues

greasy

Hair that feels "wet" to the touch. This hair type usually needs to be shampooed daily.

how to combat it

Tip 1: Try not to touch it. We know it's hard, but keep those hands off! You'll find this easier if the hair is up and out of your face. Put it in a braid, throw it up in a bun or wear a brightly colored headband.

Tip 2: Make dry shampoo your best friend. It soaks up hair oils. (For our favorites, see page 36.)

Tip 3: Avoid oils and serums. Focus on using products that have volumizing properties. (Our favorite volumizing powder: page 64).

damaged

Hair that looks dry and dull.

how to combat it

Tip 1: Limit the use of heat-styling tools. Let hair breathe by embracing your natural red strands.

Tip 2: Treat yourself to an at-home deep-conditioning treatment. Note: This may have to be done a few times, depending on how damaged your hair is.

How to Condition: Follow the RedSHAMPion Process (page 32). Apply deep conditioner to damp hair and rinse after 3 to 5 minutes. Looking for a deeper condition? Leave on for 1 hour, cover with a shower cap and apply heat to hair. This will help hair absorb the conditioner, creating shiny, healthy strands.

our "redhead friendly" favorites

$: TIGI Bed Head Urban Antidotes Recovery Conditioner

$$: Davines NOUNOU Hair Mask

Nature has thankfully provided its own ways of strengthening hair. If you do not want to break the bank, here are some ways you can enhance the health of your hair right from your kitchen.

olive oil

Our #1 favorite tip when redheads ask us, "How can my hair grow long, thick and healthy?" The natural properties in olive oil add moisture, vitality and strength to red hair and help restore smoothness, silkiness and shine. Also, it's very beneficial for the scalp because it increases blood circulation and stimulates hair growth.

How to Use: Gently heat 2 to 3 tablespoons (30 to 44 ml) of olive oil until it's warm. (Never apply boiling olive oil to your hair, you will burn your scalp!) Carefully pour on the head evenly. Brush the hair to distribute the olive oil. Use a plastic hair cap to lock in the heat and oil. Do this once or twice a week.

If you're looking for instant fullness, there are great arrays of red wigs on the market. Invest in an expensive wig for the most natural look.

avocado

Avocados are great for hydrating and nourishing the hair, and for that reason they are an ingredient in many hair products. An avocado hair mask is perfect for those with a dry scalp or dry hair.

to make an avocado hair mask, you will need

This recipe is for long hair. For short hair, use half the recipe.

+ 1 ripe avocado, pitted, peeled and mashed into a guacamole-like paste

+ 2 tablespoons (30 ml) extra-virgin olive oil

Step 1. Mix avocado with olive oil. Stir until olive oil isn't noticeable in the mixture.

Step 2. Apply mask to damp hair

Step 3. After 30 minutes, rinse off and shampoo well. Dry and enjoy your beautiful red hair.

eggs

Eggs are the best for hair growth and add shine to red locks because they are high in protein and help make the hair follicle stronger. The result? Fewer split ends and thick, strong hair.

to make an egg hair mask, you will need

+ 2 to 3 eggs

Step 1. Mix the eggs in a bowl until it thickens to a lotion texture.

Step 2. Apply throughout hair and wash out after 20 minutes.

honey

Honey gives red hair shine and strength because it has an abundance of antioxidants and vitamins. Honey nurtures the hair follicles, encouraging hair growth.

how to use

Because of its sticky texture, it's best to mix honey with water before use. Mix enough water to thin ¼ cup (60 ml) honey; the texture should have a shampoo–like appearance. Apply the mixture directly to the head to prevent a sticky mess in the hands. Apply as you would shampoo and let sit for 15 minutes. You have the option of wrapping the hair into a bun or in a plastic cap. Rinse out with warm water.

bananas

Bananas are rich in minerals and vitamins (vitamins E, C, B and A) that help to promote healthy skin and hair recovery. Tryptophan is an amino acid found in bananas, which makes it the perfect ingredient for beauty treatments. Bananas are very good for the hair and scalp because they coat dull and rough hair with vitamins, making the hair much more manageable. Regular application of bananas is also known to control dandruff and helps to soften hair.

how to use

Step 1. Mix 3 tablespoons (45 ml) of honey with a ripe banana and apply to wet hair.

Step 2. Wait 30 minutes and shampoo. This will increase the moisture content in the hair.

coconut oil

There are many benefits to using coconut oil on your hair. The reason it is so powerful is because it has protein structures that closely mimic that of our hair and skin. This means it's able to lend protein to our hair and help restore it to a certain extent. It also has moisturizing properties to balance hair moisture levels, which can add elasticity and reduce frizz.

how to use

Heat 1–2 tablespoons (15–30 ml) of coconut oil, depending on hair length. Set with a hair cap as you would with olive oil.

apple cider vinegar

Celebrity colorist, James Corbett, loves apple cider vinegar rinses to manage wild red hair. He recommends making your own by mixing two parts apple cider vinegar to one part distilled water and spritzing on dry hair after shampooing. "The vinegar brings down the pH level of the hair by closing the hair cuticle. This simple little trick can be kept in a spray bottle. It helps keep the hair shiny, less tangled and if you color your hair it helps to lock in the color."

Tip: Get a trim every 8 weeks. This will give your hair new life.

If you're a redhead "by choice," your hair is more susceptible to damage because the chemicals in hair dye strip the hair. It's essential to use deep conditioners, hair masks and avoid the use of heat and chemical-processed styling products.

Having trouble growing your hair long? Clip-in extensions are incredibly expensive, but you can make your own at a fraction of the price. Visit a local hair supply store and purchase extensions per your hair length and shade of red hair. If you can't find your exact shade, go a shade darker, not lighter. The dark effect underneath your hair will look more natural. Make sure the extensions are real human hair, as synthetic hair will not blend in well with your natural hair. They can be worn 24/7 for months and washed, brushed, straightened and curled.

to make the hair clips, you will need

+ 1 to 2 packets of hair, on a weft (do *not* buy "ponytail hair," which is loose and difficult to work with)

+ 15 to 20 wig clips

+ Sharp scissors, to cut the wefts and trim the final pieces

+ Needle and strong matching or invisible thread, to sew the wefts and clips together

Step 1: Hair comes on a long weft and is very thin. You'll want to double and/or triple it up before wearing.

Step 2: You can mess around and figure out what works best for you and your hair type, but a typical set of clip-ins would include four wide back pieces and four to six small side pieces.

Step 3: Hand sew the hair to the top of the wig clips with matching or invisible thread.

Step 4: Wig clips have combs that slide into the hair and come in a rounded shape to fit against the head. They snap shut by pressing down on the sides and open by pressing the center and pulling up on the sides. Make sure you practice opening and closing them.

Step 5: Simply clip the hair into the bottom half and sides of the head and you're done!

split ends

No one wants spilt ends, especially redheads.

how to combat them

Tip 1: When getting a haircut, make sure to tell your stylist to cut enough off so your split ends don't continue to grow.

Tip 2: Don't pick at split ends. This will only make them worse.

Tip 3: Avoid adding heat to the ends. Let them dry naturally. Bonus: Give ends a conditioner treatment by adding conditioner directly to the ends. Rinse after 5 to 10 minutes, or keep on overnight for a deep, deep treatment.

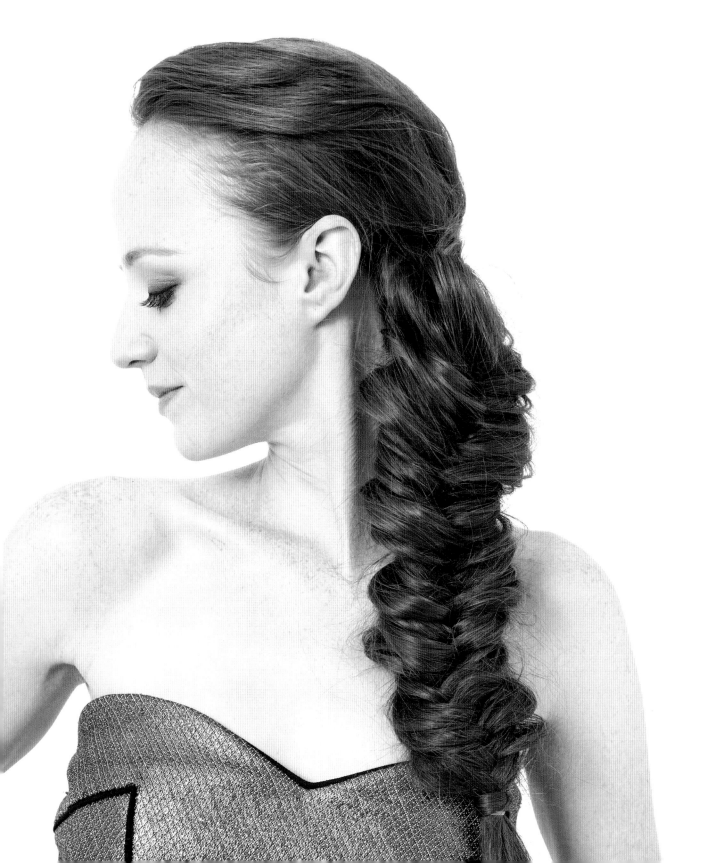

hairstyles

These are our favorite complementary hairstyles for redheads.

redhead braids

The foundation of a beautiful and flawless braid is all in the preparation. Brush hair until smooth and apply a thin layer of styling creme from roots to ends to prevent any flyaways. If the roots need a refresh, use a dry shampoo. A braid is a great style between shampoos!

the fishtail braid

Tools: Tail comb and redhead hair ties

1. Create desired part and gather the hair at the nape of the neck.

2. Split ponytail into two equal sections.

3. Take a thin section of hair from the outside of the right and cross it over to the inside of left.

4. Take a small section from the outside of the left and cross it over to the inside of the right.

5. Continue working from right to left until you have completed your braid.

Taking smaller sections of hair will deliver a more intricate look.
Be sure to keep a firm hold so the braid is tight. For a more playful look,
loosen up the braid after it's completed.

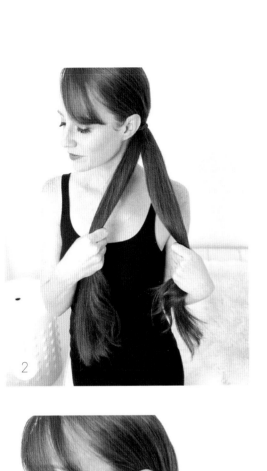

2

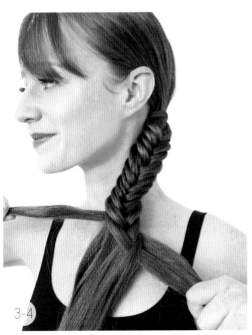

3-4

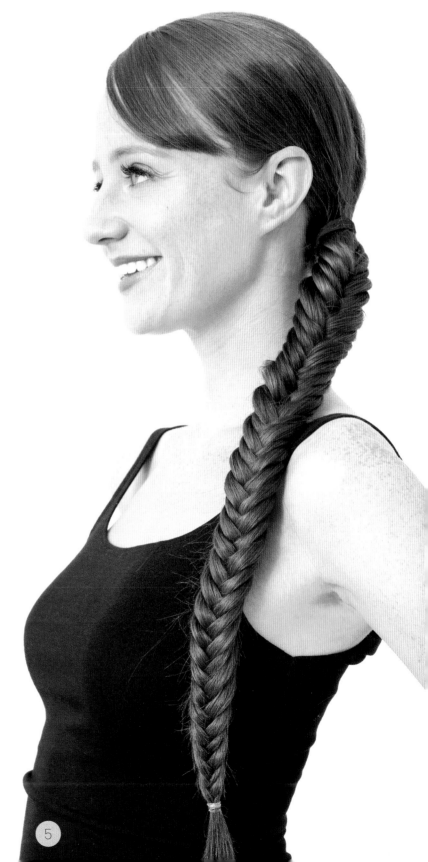

5

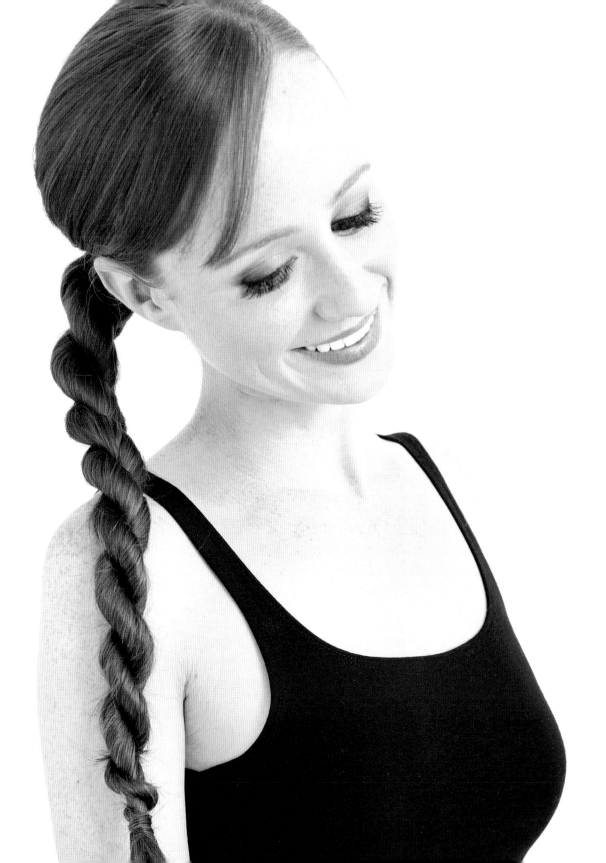

the basic rope braid

Tools: Tail comb and two redhead hair ties

1. Gather hair in a ponytail and secure with redhead hair tie.

2. Divide hair into two equal sections.

3. Twist both sections of hair to the right four times and then cross the right section of hair up and over the left.

4. Repeat until the braid is complete. Secure with a redhead hair tie.

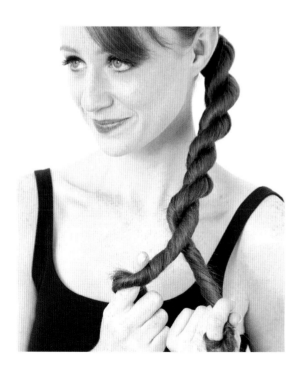 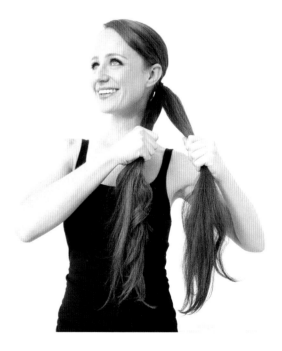

the crown braid—invisible/visible

Tools: Tail comb and one redhead hair tie

1. Create a diagonal section on the top of the head where the braid will begin.

2. Pick up a small triangle of hair at the base of that section and divide into three parts.

3. Begin to braid by bringing the right section to center then the left to center.

4. As you repeat, marry small sections of hair from the right and left side into the braid. Work around the head until you reach a desired stopping point or travel all around the head for a beautiful updo. Secure with redhead hair tie.

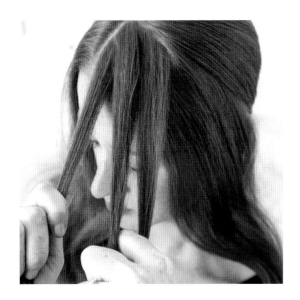 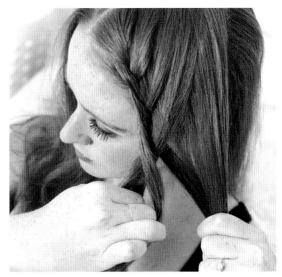

Crossing sections underneath one another will create the visible look, while crossing sections over one another will create the invisible braid.

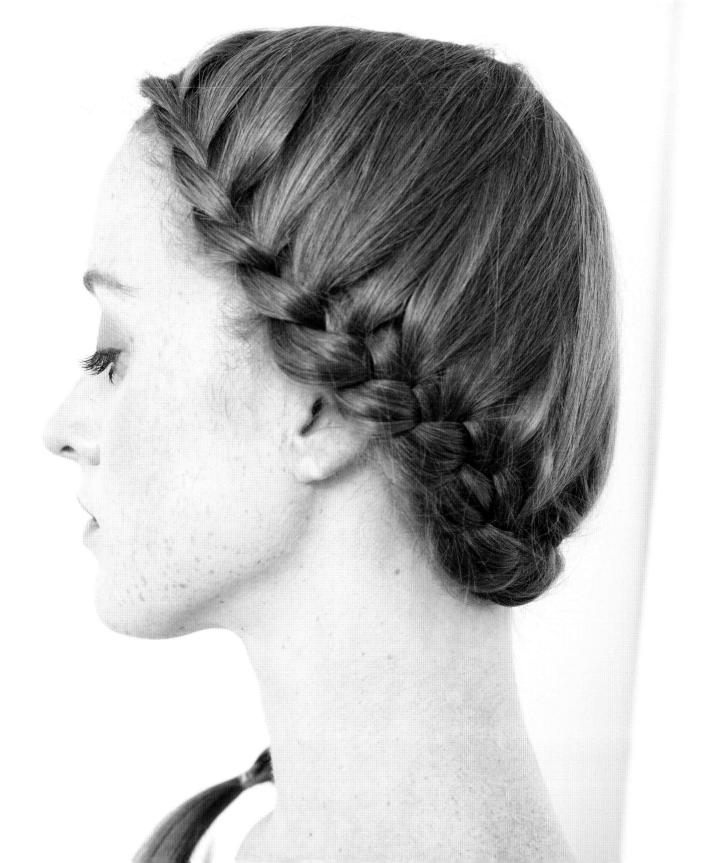

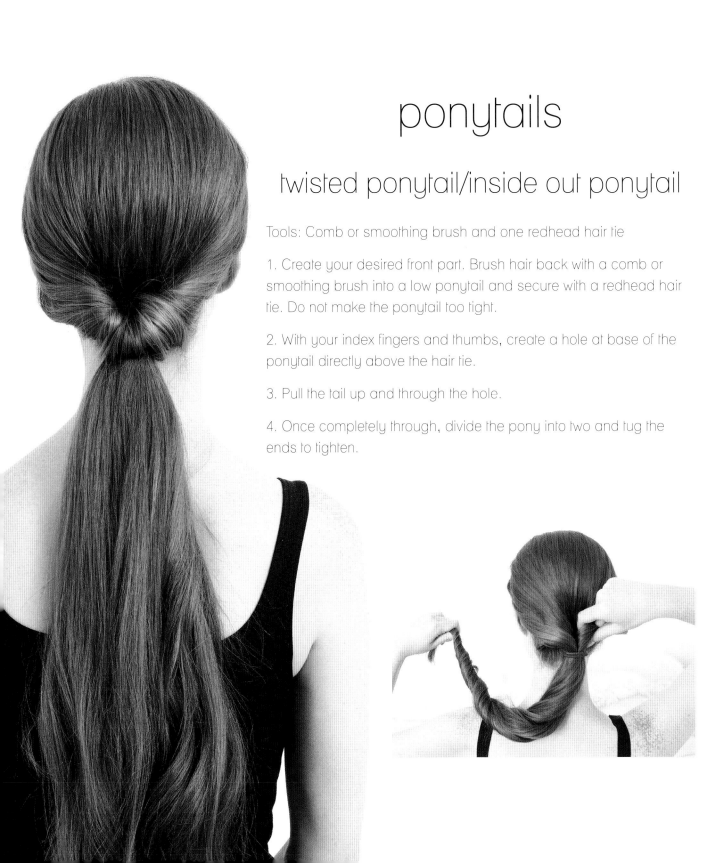

ponytails

twisted ponytail/inside out ponytail

Tools: Comb or smoothing brush and one redhead hair tie

1. Create your desired front part. Brush hair back with a comb or smoothing brush into a low ponytail and secure with a redhead hair tie. Do not make the ponytail too tight.

2. With your index fingers and thumbs, create a hole at base of the ponytail directly above the hair tie.

3. Pull the tail up and through the hole.

4. Once completely through, divide the pony into two and tug the ends to tighten.

the perfect ponytail

Tools: Boar bristle brush, tail comb, one redhead hair tie, two redhead bobby pins and hairspray

1. Create a bungee cord with two bobby pins and one hair tie by inserting a bobby pin at each separate end of the hair tie. Set aside.

2. Brush hair to center back of head, using a boar bristle brush for optimal smoothness, and hold the ponytail at the base with one hand.

3. Use the bungee cord to insert one bobby pin on a vertical angle to the left side of the ponytail base, and then wrap the hair tie around the base clockwise until taut.

4. Insert the second bobby pin into the base of ponytail until secure.

5. Take a small section of hair from the bottom of the left side and spray it heavily with hairspray. Wrap it clockwise around the ponytail spritzing with hairspray with every new layer until the hair is wrapped securely.

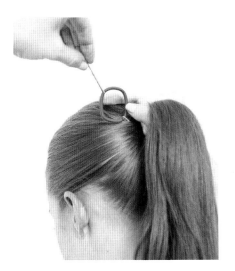
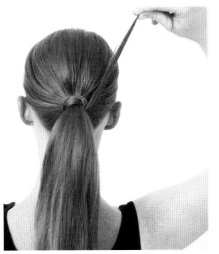
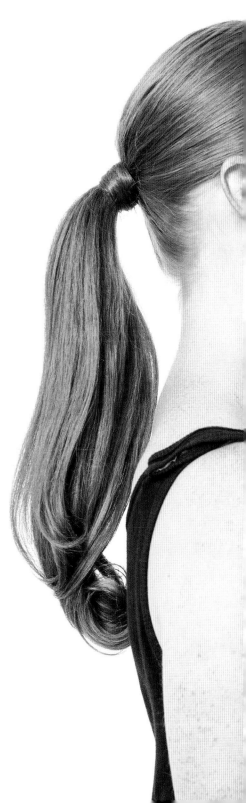

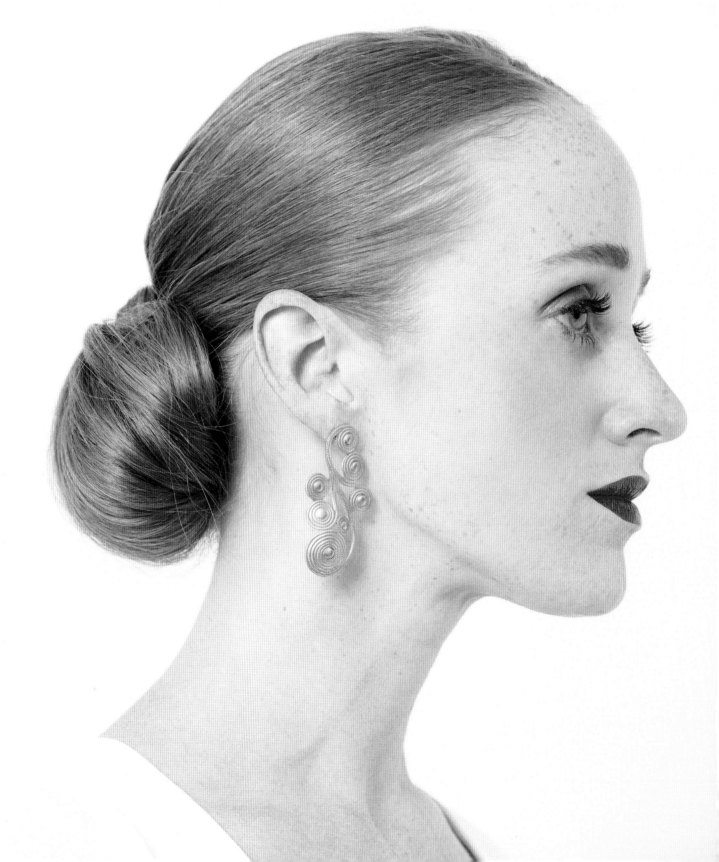

other favorite hairstyles
chignon

Tools: Brush, tail comb, one redhead hair tie, six redhead bobby pins and hairspray

1. Create the Perfect Ponytail (page 101).

2. Roll the tail ends of hair under and up until they meet the base of the ponytail.

3. Tuck chin down to create tension and secure the rolled ends into the base of ponytail with bobby pins on a vertical upward slant. Spray with hairspray to complete the look.

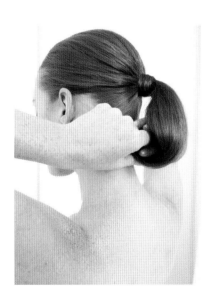 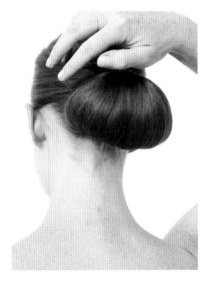 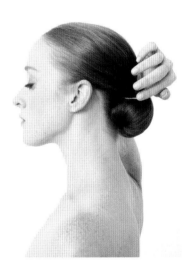

bun

Classy Look: Use the Redhead Bun Maker to create a classic, beautiful bun.

Tools: One Redhead Bun Maker, one redhead hair tie and one or two bobby pins

1. You will need to match the color of the bun maker to your red hair as close as possible.

2. Hold hair into a ponytail. Bear in mind that where you position this will determine your bun's final position, so aim high if you are wanting a top knot or ballerina-style bun.

3. Use the bun maker and thread ponytail through its middle.

4. Find the center of your ponytail where it is pulled through the bun maker and spread the hair around to cover the sponge. You can easily feel where the doughnut is still poking through, so just use your hands to smooth the hair round evenly until you're happy.

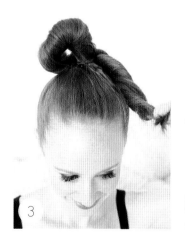
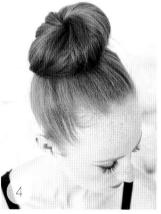
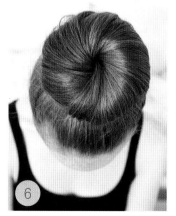
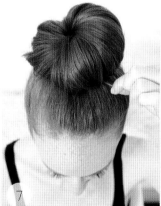

5. With one hand on the center of the bun (to keep the main shape in place), slowly start to wind the end of the hair in a circular a motion around the bun maker.

6. As you wrap it around, you'll find it naturally tucks in under the bun, so just work your way around, keeping the bun tight (and making sure that the bun is still smooth and fully covered).

7. Use a redhead bobby pin to secure the hair wrapped around the bottom of the bun. Depending on the thickness of your hair, you may need another redhead bobby pin to secure the look. At this point you can make the bun as neat or messy as you like.

Messy Look: We love the look of irregularities and lots of frizziness when red hair is wrapped in a messy bun. Hold clean hair into a ponytail at the top of the head and wrap the hair into a bun–like shape. Secure with a redhead bobby pin or two (depending on the thickness of your hair) at the bottom of the bun.

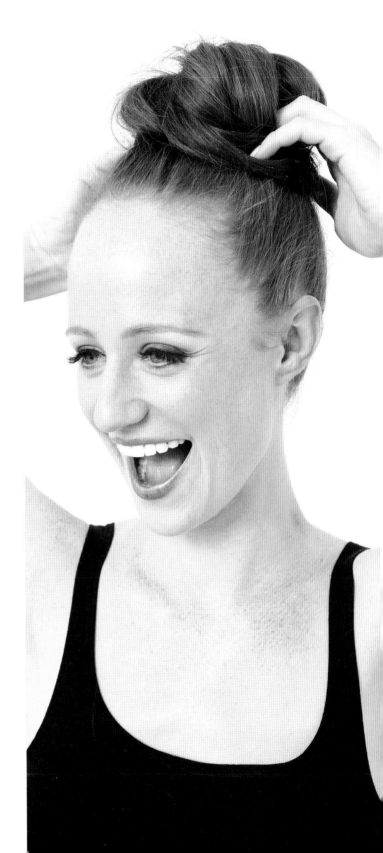

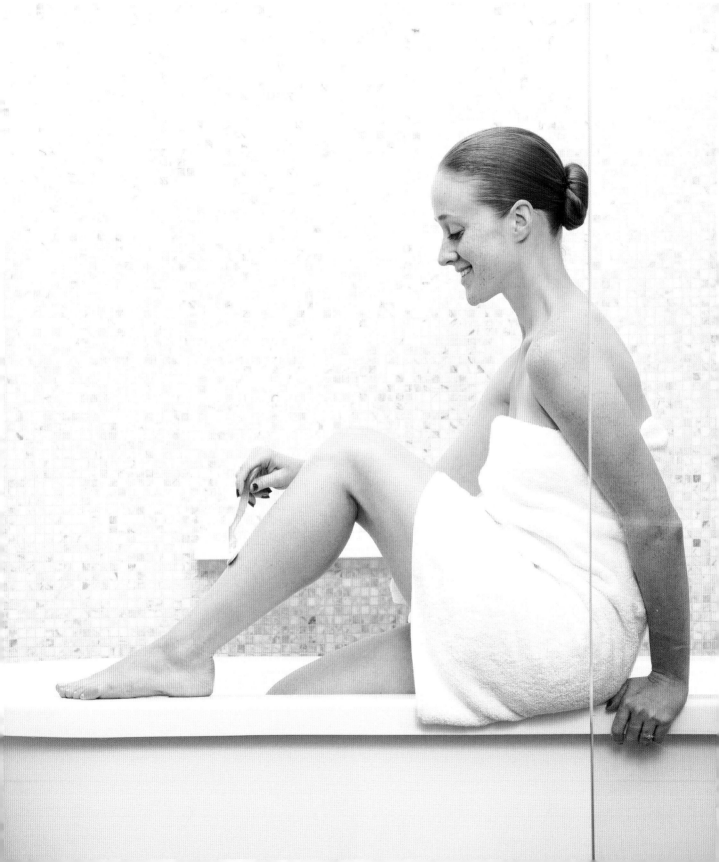

shaving and waxing

Many redheads with sensitive skin have to be careful when it comes to hair removal. This type of skin is the most tender, causing hair cuticles to have a higher reaction when being pulled and removed. To avoid razor bumps, rashes, redness and irritation, we suggest the following "redhead friendly" tips to make hair happy and healthy:

1. Shave every other day or every two days, depending on how the skin reacts to the blade when the hairs aren't that long.

2. Always shave toward the end of your shower. This will give your pores time to open, avoiding ingrown hairs, redness and irritation.

3. Waxing is a great option that saves a lot of time in the shower. We highly recommend making sure your esthetician is using sensitive-skin wax.

4. Use an all-natural sensitive-skin shaving cream to help your razor do its job. It's also a great way to keep track of where you already shaved. Our "redhead friendly" favorite: Alba Botanica Very Emolliant Natural Moisturizing Cream Shave. After shaving, don't forget to apply a body oil or moisturizer. This will hydrate the pores and eliminate any ingrown hairs.

5. Coconut oil is another great option for shaving cream. Simply apply the same way you would shaving cream.

6. Ran out of shaving cream? Shampoo, conditioner and lotion are all great alternatives to use.

7. Opt for a five-blade razor to ensure a smooth, even shave. We love Schick Intuition Naturals Sensitive Care Razor.

8. Getting a bikini wax? Choose hard wax over strips because hard wax is gentler on sensitive skin.

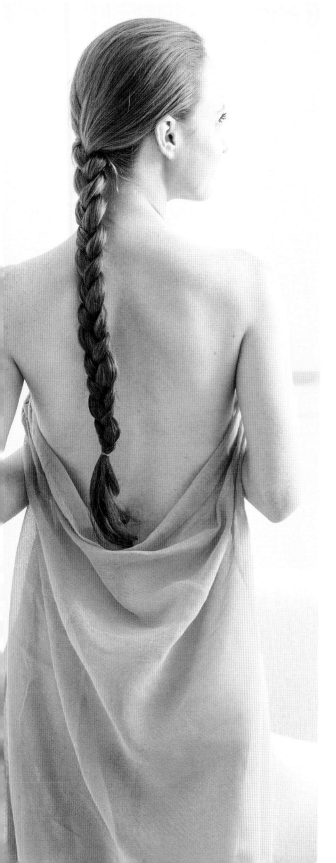

9. Do you have problems with bumps on your legs from shaving? Do the bumps resemble bug bites and begin to itch and sometimes hurt? If you stop shaving, do they not go away? If you've answered yes to any or all of these questions, you might be allergic to the metal or nickel in your razor. Here are a few quick tips to make sure you're living a nickel-free razor life:

+ Get tested by a doctor to see if you are in fact allergic to nickel.

+ Use a razor where the metal part is only in the blade and the rest is plastic. Sometimes, the metal around the blade can comprise pure nickel, and that in itself can cause extreme irritation.

+ Stop using your razor if you suspect a nickel allergy. The irritation will become worse and worse.

10. Threading is an ancient method of hair removal originating in Central Asia and India. In threading, a thin thread is doubled and then twisted. It is then rolled over areas of unwanted hair, plucking the hair at the follicle level. Unlike tweezing, where single hairs are pulled out one at a time, threading can remove short lines of hair. It is a great hair removal choice for redheads because it is nonabrasive to the skin. But make sure to consult with your local threading salon. There have been cases where the threading was unsanitary because those who did the threading kept the thread in their mouth as they shape.

11. Redheads cannot get laser hair removal.

haircut advice

I (Stephanie) have had the worst luck with haircuts. When Adrienne was five and I was three, she used kitchen scissors to cut off (mostly) all of my hair. We laugh about it now, but I was definitely scared. It took years for my hair to grow back. Then, when I was in grade school and already incredibly insecure about my red hair, I went to get a haircut and walked out with way too many inches cut off. It was shorter than a bob, and I cried for days.

The best haircut advice is to go to a consultation and bring photos of your desired look. As you're describing what you want, make sure the stylist is listening to you. If you want long hair, tell the stylist you're growing it out and be very specific about how much you want cut off. It isn't unusual to have a hairstylist suggest something else, but if they're pushing you, go to a new stylist.

Nick Arrojo, owner and founder of ARROJO salons in NYC, has some good advice on the importance of the right haircut for a redhead: "I think there are so many advertisements, so many *so called* experts giving advice and so many new miracle products claiming to cure anything that ails you, that women tend to get confused and forget about the most important things: healthy hair is the number one goal because it is the shiniest and most lustrous and to focus on getting a haircut that complements the beautiful features of your face, like the eyes, cheekbones, neck and chin."

With that said, here are Nick's guidelines for each type of face shape:

oval

Considered the most balanced face shape. Those with an oval face can wear any type of cut, so be adventurous! Choose details that emphasize your best features. Great eyes? Sport a fringe. Beautiful, slender neck? Go for something short to show it off. One of my favorite looks for this face shape is a long layered cut with a side part, styled into waves, with the short side of the part pushed behind the ear and the long side tumbling forward, creating face-framing asymmetry.

round

The face is widest at the cheekbones. If you are going to wear bangs, opt for side-swept bangs and avoid blunt or straight-across bangs as these will emphasize the rounded width of the face. If you are going to wear a bob, make it slightly A-line, which will slenderize the face. If you are going to wear longer hair with layers, always begin the layering below the chin.

3

square

The face is widest at the forehead and the jaw. Avoid chin-length cuts as they emphasize the squareness of the jaw. Go for cuts with softness and texture to offset the strength of a square face. If wearing hair long, asymmetrical and short-to-long styles will help to balance the face. Razor cuts are a great option as they create fluid softness in the hair.

heart

The heart-shape face is perfect for bobs that reach the jaw or chin area because these shapes will give the illusion of width where the face is most narrow. Longer side bangs will help visually slenderize the forehead area, which is the widest part of this shape. If going for a shorter look, something asymmetrical can also help slim down the forehead area and highlight the cheekbones. Long hair? Have layering or face framing begin below jaw.

oblong

To keep face looking full and not too slender, go for layered styles that can be styled to add width and volume through the sides, which will add life to the face.

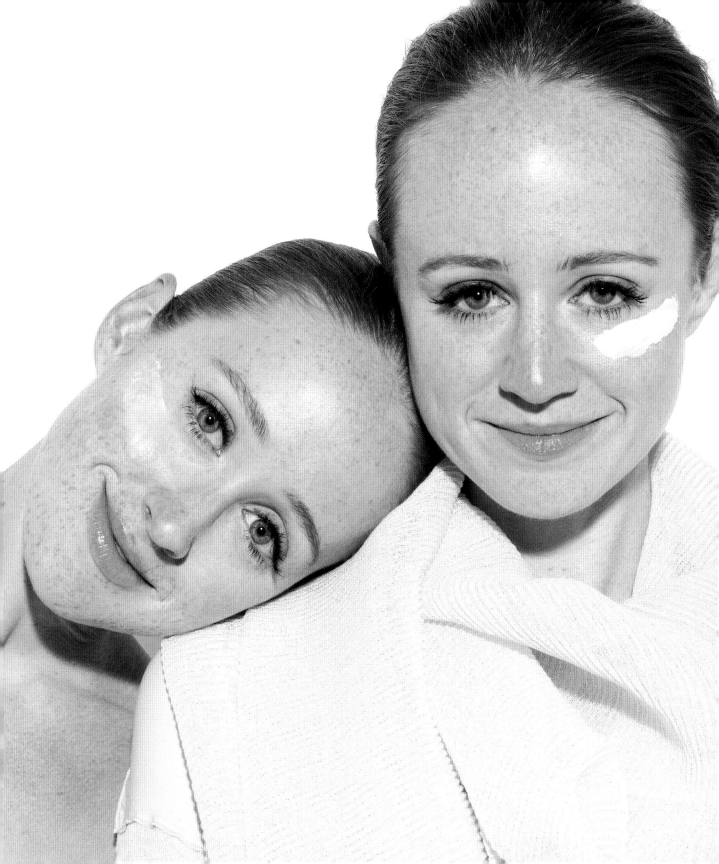

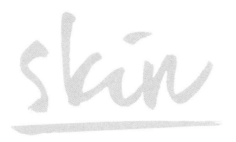

skin

The skin is sometimes the most challenging part about being a redhead. In most cases, redheads have very sensitive skin, and when puberty occurs or experimentation with makeup begins, a redhead's reaction might be completely different from that of her blonde or brunette friends. When you have sensitive skin, which can result in rosacea or acne, it takes a long time to conquer problems for perfect-looking skin.

As a teenager, I (Adrienne) suffered from acne, especially on my face and back, and still battle with bumps from sensitive skin breakouts on my chest and arms on a daily basis. It took Stephanie and I testing hundreds of products and breaking out a million times to finally get our daily regimen down to a science. Thankfully, you will not have to do the same.

Over the years, I've learned that when friends are sharing their favorite makeup products or tanning at the beach, a redhead always has to make a conscious effort to love her skin the way it is naturally. You have only one skin, so treat it with care.

Stephanie had a hard time accepting her freckles. She spent her teenage years searching for how she could get rid of them and invested a ton of money in foundations to make her "sun kisses" disappear.

We both hated our pale skin. We use to ask each other, "Why can't we be tan like our friends and family?" Yes, the majority of our family has olive skin and brown hair! I used to wear dark foundation to make my skin look tan, but looking back, it looked orange and fake. I also used to go spray tanning two to three times a week to prolong my orange glow.

Sooner or later, we both looked in the mirror and thought, "What are we doing?"

Now, we love our red hair, freckles and fair skin. We understand every redhead insecurity that exists and have pushed through it, and we've had plenty of laughs in the end. We've learned that different is not only good, but it's what everyone should strive for.

Why fit in when you were put on this earth to make a statement?

"A redhead's skin is usually very sun sensitive, fair and usually sensitive to products. Sensitive skin is genetic, just like a redhead's red hair is genetic. That's just the way it is. Go for products that say 'for gentle skin' on the label. Avoid scrubs, which abrade the skin and cause irritation. Gentle peels, serums with vitamin C and peptides for face and eyes work on wrinkles. Laser treatments are available in gentle treatment levels and are highly recommended."

—Dr. Dennis Gross, dermatologist and creator of Dr. Dennis Gross Skincare

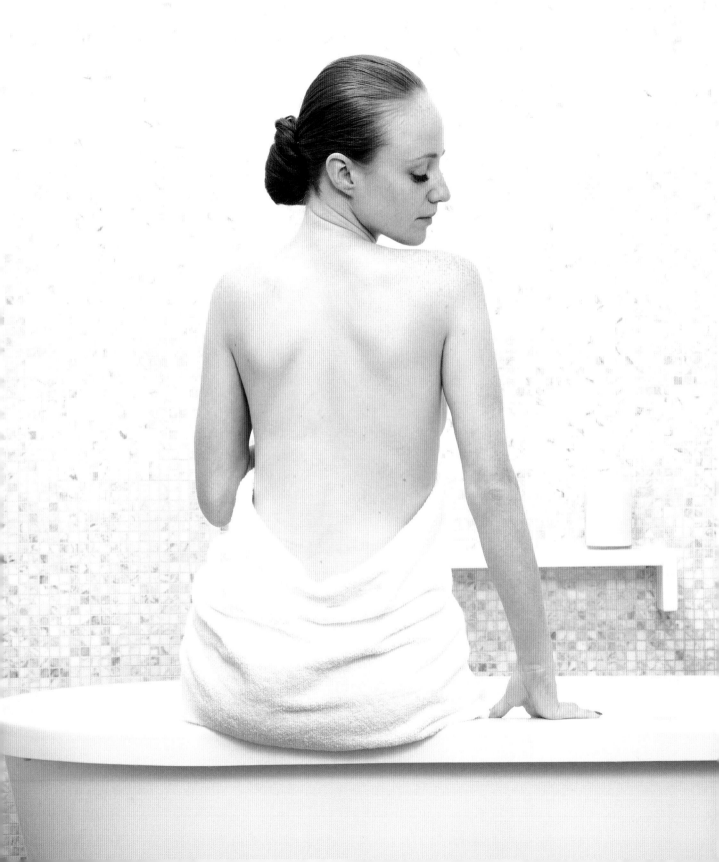

skin types

dry

This skin type feels tight, flaky and sometimes itchy. It can be painful and lead to conditions like eczema. This uncomfortable feeling stems from a lack of moisture and is the opposite of oily. Redheads with dry skin must moisturize frequently and use products with natural-based oils to give life to the skin.

oily

If you feel like you have to wash your skin again shortly after washing it, you might experience oily skin. This type of skin has an excess amount of oils, especially within the T-zone (the forehead, nose, lip area and chin), because of the oil glands on the forehead, nose and chin. It's important for redheads with oily skin to invest in a quality moisturizer that gently removes oil and doesn't strip the skin.

combo

A blend of both oily and dry. Most experience oily skin on the T-zone and dryness on the cheeks. It's important for this skin type to spot treat, meaning you might need lighter products for the T-zone and a heavy moisturizer on the cheeks.

sensitive skin

This is the most common skin type among redheads. It usually stems from a bad reaction to cosmetics and/or skincare products. A woman with sensitive skin is accustomed to the feeling of itching and irritation and is commonly allergic to certain ingredients in skin products (like heavy chemicals such as sulfates and parabens). These types of ingredients can cause mild to extreme skin irritation. The flare-ups can even be in the form of rosacea, an inflammatory skin condition that causes redness and bumps on the cheeks, chin, nose and forehead. Many redheads face skin sensitivity in the sun and heat. It's best, and highly recommended, to wear plenty of sunscreen and use sulfate-free and paraben-free products.

How do you know if you have sensitive skin?

Does your skin become red to the touch? Do you have visible capillaries? If you answered "yes" to either of these questions, you have sensitive skin.

5

normal

This type of skin is not too dry and not too oily. It's a normal skin tone, without acne, sun damage or large pores. It is usually even and doesn't need much makeup. This is the rarest skin type among women (and redheads), because most experience some type of oily, dry, sensitive or combo.

Both Adrienne and Stephanie have combo and sensitive skin.

"redhead friendly" skin products for the face

(1)

cleanser

A cleanser is a facial care product that is used to remove makeup, dead skin, oil, dirt and other types of pollutants from the face. It helps to unclog pores and prevent skin conditions such as blackheads and acne.

Refer to chart on pages 130–131 for cleanser recommendations for each skin type.

gel vs. cream cleansers

Gel cleansers are best for redheads with oily skin since they are formulated to strip excess oils from the face. Cream cleansers are intended to add moisture to your skin.

"redhead friendly" tip: Redheads should always use a cleanser that is made for sensitive skin. Many cleansers designed without sensitive skin in mind can be harsh and cause breakouts.

Did you know? There are more pores on the face than anywhere else on your body. This is why the face is very sensitive, and for redheads, who have thinner skin than anyone else, it's imperative to pamper the skin to maintain the glow and keep it safe. Make sure never to wash your face with hot water and always moisturize.

toner

Toner is usually the second step in the face-washing regimen and comes in a spray or pump. After washing your face, gently apply toner to the face with a cotton pad. You'll instantly feel a sense of tingling throughout your skin—this is a sign that the toner is doing its job! Toners moisturize, wash away any oil or dirt you may have missed while cleansing and tighten any opened pores.

"redhead friendly" tip: Make sure to use a toner that is alcohol-free. Alcohol is extremely drying, and a redhead's skin can be stripped and suffer as a result. Using alcohol-free witch hazel is a great option for a toner because the natural ingredients remove excess oils from the face and minimizes pores.

exfoliator

Exfoliation removes dead skin cells, leaving redhead skin radiant and smooth. Typically, an exfoliator's main ingredients are raw sugar, sea salt, ground almonds, walnuts, seeds or other grainy components.

"redhead friendly" tip: It's recommended that redheads exfoliate their face and body only once or twice a week maximum. Excessive exfoliation can cause breakouts, bumps, rashes and extreme skin sensitivity. Want softer lips? Exfoliate them once or twice a week. This will remove any dry skin that may have surfaced on the lips. Our favorite "redhead friendly" product is Fresh Sugar Lip Polish.

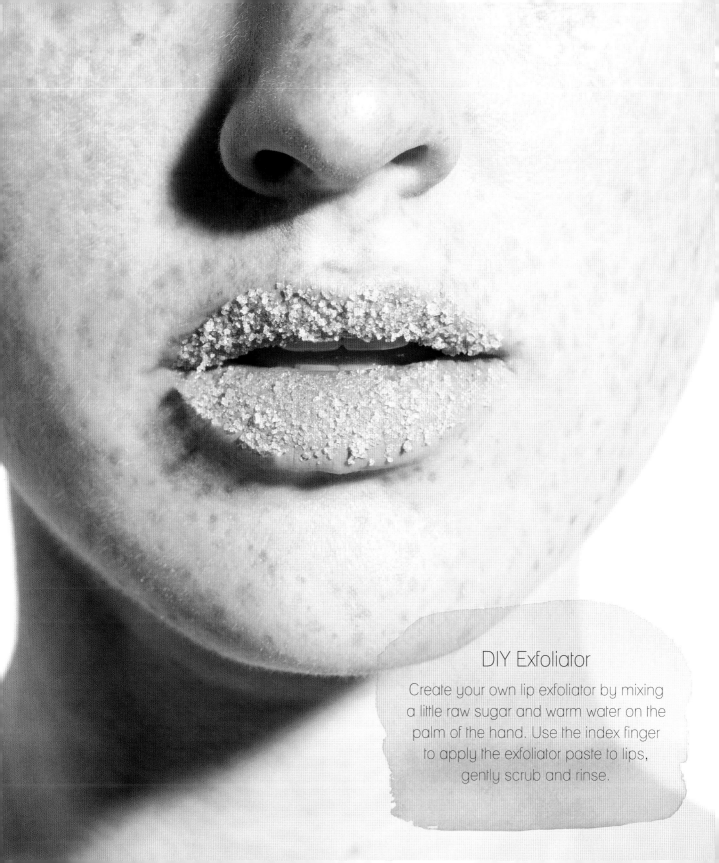

DIY Exfoliator

Create your own lip exfoliator by mixing
a little raw sugar and warm water on the
palm of the hand. Use the index finger
to apply the exfoliator paste to lips,
gently scrub and rinse.

daytime moisturizer

Redhead skin needs TLC. A daytime moisturizer hydrates the skin, leaving you ready to conquer the day.

"redhead friendly" tips

+ Don't forget to apply moisturizer on the neck, and always apply with an upward motion, as you never want to pull the skin down. If you suffer from dry areas on your face (mainly on the cheeks) and feel a sense of stiffness after applying a moisturizer, consider a new all-natural moisturizer.

+ Coconut oil is a great moisturizer for redheads because it soothes and protects sensitive skin without the use of harsh chemicals. To use, scoop out a chunk at a time and rub it along your skin. The cool chunks will melt as they interact with the warmth of your skin.

"Use a light moisturizer if you have oily skin. Sensitive-skin redheads should use moisturizers with a lot of herbs and chamomile in them."

—Susan Ciminelli, owner of Susan Ciminelli Beauty Clinic
and holistic skincare expert

5

serum

Face serums are lightweight moisturizers that penetrate deeper to deliver active ingredients to the skin. They're great for redhead skin because they regenerate moisture without leaving skin greasy.

"redhead friendly" tip: Serums will moisturize only to a minimal extent, so make sure to use them in conjunction with heavier moisturizers. If you have a chronic skin condition such as eczema or rosacea, serums may aggravate it.

6

oils

We love oils. Period. They can be a blend of plant-based oils, and they penetrate easily into the skin, causing ultimate moisture. Apply to damp face and neck. We suggest an all-natural face oil so it won't clog the pores. Once applied, don't worry about the oil excess, it will eventually dissolve into your skin.

"redhead friendly" tip: In most instances, redheads have oily and sensitive skin. Many think they cannot use face oils because it will make the skin even oilier, but it's actually quite the opposite. The skin is oily in the first place because it is trying to make more oil. So, when you apply oils to the skin, you'll notice the skin appear more even and less sensitive.

our "redhead friendly" favorites

Argan oil • Rose hip oil • Jojoba oil

Lavender oil • Olive oil

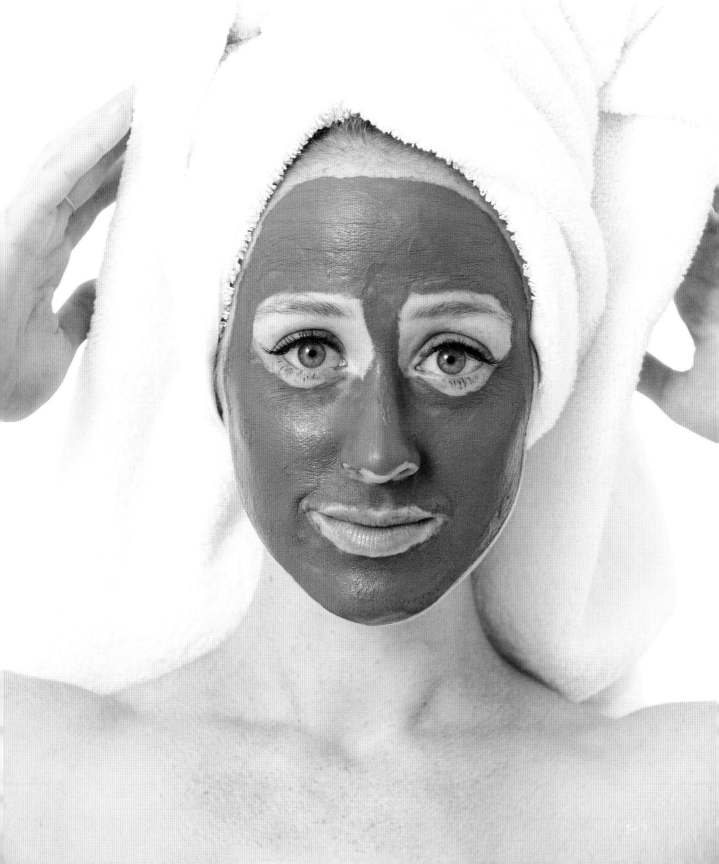

masks

They unclog pores, draw up impurities that hide beneath the skin and help maintain a glowing, effortless complexion. We love giving ourselves a complete face mask once a week. It gives us an excuse for a little me time, while also treating the skin to some pampering.

"redhead friendly" tips

+ Apply mask for 5 to 10 minutes then rinse. If your skin needs some extra love, apply the mask before bed and rinse in the morning. Have a pimple or two? Apply mask directly to pimple for spot treatment.

+ We love keeping our face masks in the fridge so they're cool when we apply them to our skin.

our "redhead friendly" favorites

$: Origins Drink Up! 10 Minute Mask to Quench Skin's Thirst

$$: Tata Harper Resurfacing Mask

"A great DIY mask should be yogurt based because yogurt is a natural anti-inflammatory. I recommend mixing a cup of yogurt with honey and strawberries for a pure tightening, hydrating and soothing mask. Treat dryness with shea butter, cocoa butter, avocado oil and almond oil. They keep the skin super hydrated without clogging the pores."

—Joanna Vargas, founder of Joanna Vargas Salon
and Skin Care in NYC

night cream

Nighttime is the best time to hydrate the skin so you can wake up looking even more fabulous. Applying a night cream before heading to bed is a great way to moisturize and rejuvenate the skin.

"redhead friendly" tip: The skin actually repairs itself while you're sleeping. While the skin is repairing, the night cream will be working hard to keep the skin looking ageless, too.

eye cream

The skin around the eye is the thinnest skin on the face so it's very important to protect and hydrate at all times. Plus, a great eye cream can prevent wrinkles and fine lines.

"redhead friendly" tip: Using only one finger, pat the product gently around the eye. The less friction around the eye, the better!

our "redhead friendly" favorites

$: Simple Skincare Revitalizing Eye Roll-On

$$: PCA Skin Ideal Complex Revitalizing Eye Gel

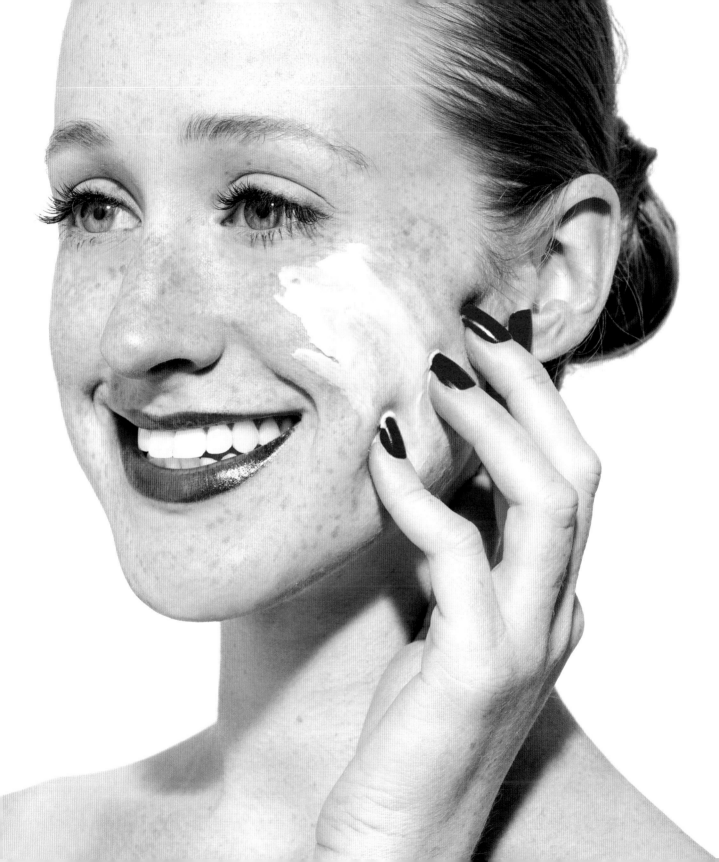

spot treatment

Spot treatment, also known as pimple cream, can be used on any blemish or area of the skin that may have a pimple or two. Simply dab on the problem area and let sit on the skin for two to three hours.

"redhead friendly" tip: Don't touch or pick pimples! It will only make them worse and could create scarring.

our "redhead friendly" favorites

$: Clinique Acne Solutions Clinical Clearing Gel

$$: Susan Ciminelli Sea Clay Mask (Instead of a mask, we use it as a spot treatment.)

peels

Peels can brighten up the face, leaving skin smoother and more youthful. Peels are intended to reduce pore size and remove (or peel) the damaged outer layer of skin. A peel can be done at home or by an esthetician.

"redhead friendly" tip: BEWARE! Whether you're using an at-home peel or getting a professional peel, make sure it is 100% natural to refrain from redness and irritation.

our "redhead friendly" favorite

$: Dr. Dennis Gross Alpha Beta Peel

face mists

Spritz and you're off! Face mists are a great way to add an instant burst of moisture to the skin. Spray onto clean face and bring with you to reapply throughout the day. Also great for setting makeup.

"redhead friendly" tip: Stick to a mist that is all natural and alcohol-free.

our "redhead friendly" favorite

$$$: Fresh Rose Marigold Floral Water

daily skin regimens for the face

redhead daily skin regimen

	dry	oily	combo dry + oily
morning	Cleanser: Susan Ciminelli Algae Deep Cleanse Moisturizer: Clinique Dramatically Different Moisturizing Lotion+ Face Serum: Thesis Organic Face Serum Lullaby for Dry Skin Moisturizer: Josie Maran Argan Daily Moisturizer SPF 47	Cleanser: La Roche-Posay Effaclar Purifying Foaming Gel Cleanser Toner: Avene Gentle Toner Moisturizer: (MALIN + GOETZ) Vitamin E Face Moisturizer Face Oil: Susan Ciminelli Oil Control Formula or Clarins Lotus Face Treatment Oil Oil Pads: Desert Essence Natural Tea Tree Oil Facial Cleansing Pads or boscia Clear Complexion Blotting Linens	Cleanser: boscia Detoxifying Black Cleanser Toner: Fresh Rose Floral Toner Serum: Clinique Pore Refining Solutions Correcting Serum Moisturizer: Juice Beauty SPF 30 Oil-Free Moisturizer Apply the Serum and Moisturizer heavily on the cheeks where dry skin usually occurs with combo skin.
night	Use the same cleanser, face serum and oil as you did in the morning, but use a night cream to keep skin heavily moisturized throughout the night. Our Favorite: Ahava Time To Hydrate Night Replenisher	Remember, it's important to use many oils when the skin is oily. It keeps the skin balanced and youthful. At night, use a heavier moisturizer designed for oily skin and one to two face oils of your choice. Our Favorite: Kiehl's Ultra Facial Oil-Free Gel Cream (for Normal to Oily Skin)	Follow the same morning skin regimen for combo skin at night. You may choose to opt for a moisturizer without SPF. Our Favorite: Mario Badescu Seaweed Night Cream

	sensitive	normal
	most common for redheads	neither dry nor oily
morning	Simply splash lukewarm water on the skin and apply a light oil. Sensitive skin does not like to be washed frequently, and too much cleansing can cause breakouts and rashes. Our Favorite Daytime Oils and Serum: Aesop Fabulous Face Oil Indie Lee Squalane Facial Oil Korres Wild Rose Face and Eye Serum	This skin type does not require much maintenance, but you should still take care of it. Cleanser: Burt's Bees Soap Bark & Chamomile Deep Cleansing Cream Toner: Aveda Green Science Replenishing Toner, use occasionally Serum: Origins Original Skin Renewal Serum with Willowherb
night	Cleanser: REN Evercalm Gentle Cleansing Milk Serum: Use ones recommended for daytime. Moisturizer: Susan Ciminelli Calming Cream Face Oil: Use ones recommended for daytime.	Follow the morning skin regimen. You may choose a heavier moisturizer without SPF. Our Favorite: Weleda Iris Hydrating Facial Lotion

skin regimens for the body

1

natural deodorant

Have you been troubled by red bumps in your armpits? Do they seem to get worse after you apply antiperspirant? Chances are, you are not using the right deodorant. The best deodorants for redheads with sensitive skin should be free of harsh chemicals such as aluminum chlorohydrate and should also be paraben- and fragrance-free.

our "redhead friendly" favorites

$: Salve: Schmidt's Natural Deodorant—Lavender & Sage

$: Stick: Kiss My Face No White Marks-Liquid Rock Roll-On-Patchouli

body oils

Oils are a great option if you do not like to use lotions as a moisturizer. We recently started using body oils and notice a significant difference. Our skin is effortlessly softer. Apply oils within three minutes of getting out of the shower for maximum absorption.

our "redhead friendly" favorites

$$: S.W. BASICS Body Oil

$$$: Tata Harper Revitalizing Body Oil

3

body lotion

Body lotion is a must, especially during the winter. Apply lotion immediately after showering. This will give the lotion the ability to come in contact with some of the water on the skin in order to achieve extra hydration. Never forget to apply lotion on the neck, elbows and ankles. These three areas tend to get overlooked and can become very dry, very fast. Also, make sure your lotion is 100% natural. This will ensure your skin does not become irritated once applied.

our "redhead friendly" favorites

$: Alba Botanica Very Emollient Body Lotion, Unscented Original

$$: Egyptian Magic All Purpose Skin Cream

body scrubs/exfoliators

Using body scrubs is a way to remove dead skin cells and leave skin feeling super soft. We recommend exfoliating once or twice a week. Choose a sugar scrub that is free of harmful ingredients (which can strip the skin) and contains natural fragrances if scented. We love coffee and sugar scrubs. They work well with sensitive skin and do not leave skin itchy and irritated. If you happen to have itchy skin after the use of a scrub, try one that is unscented. Itchiness can happen when your skin reacts to fragrances in the product.

our "redhead friendly" favorites

$: Hugo Naturals Soothing Sea Fennel & Passionflower Sea Salt & Sugar Scrub

$$: Pacifica Kona Coffee & Sugar Detox Whole Body Scrub

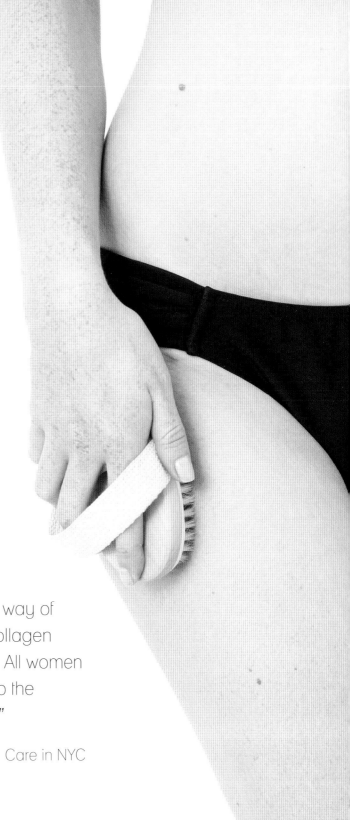

dry brushing

Purchase an all-natural (not synthetic) bristle brush with a long handle in order to reach those not-so-easy areas around your body.

For overall circulation, always brush in a circular motion. Your lymph flows toward the heart, so you're going to want to make sure you're brushing toward that area. Don't dry brush on your face or any areas of your body that are prone to sensitivity. Don't rub too hard. Gentle circular motions are best.

Always end dry brushing with a few pumps of moisturizer and big glass of water. This ensures you're clearing away any toxins just released and gives your digestive system a little healthy kick.

"Dry brushing is a great old-fashioned way of getting rid of cellulite and increasing collagen production and elasticity all over the body. All women should do this because it helps keep the body beach ready as you age."

—Joanna Vargas, founder of Joanna Vargas Skin Care in NYC

seasonal skin care

As the seasons change, so should your skincare regime. Think of it like this: would you want to wear the same oversized, chunky sweater during fall, winter, spring and summer? No way! Your skin is the same way. You don't want to use a heavy, winter moisturizer in the summer months. Redheads should be conscious of giving the skin what it needs. And trust us, your skin will thank you.

spring and summer

Use a light moisturizer with an SPF. Gel-like cleansers work best. Serums and oils should still be worn during the warmer months. Depending on where you live, your skin is probably less dry in the spring and summer, so it's safe to exfoliate the body and face once or twice a week.

fall and winter

Use heavier moisturizers with an SPF. Yes, sunscreen protection is 365 days a year! Use serums and oils. Keep exfoliation down to one or two times a month, no more than that because you do not want to create dry, itchy patches. Apply a heavier moisturizer.

Change pillowcases more often than your sheets. We recommend at least once a week because buildup can occur that may cause breakouts. Make sure you're using an all-natural detergent too!

top "redhead friendly" tips for conquering…

1

rosacea

Many fair-skinned people, like redheads, suffer from rosacea. This chronic, inflammatory skin condition affects an estimated 16 million Americans, and one of its most common (and often frustrating) symptoms is persistent facial redness. Most redheads (with rosacea or not) are already accustomed to being super picky about beauty products, making sure they do not have heavy perfumes and that they are designed for sensitive skin. The right beauty products can help reduce redness and bumps caused by rosacea, and they can also minimize irritation and soothe skin.

1. *Prime face and any problem areas.* As a first step in applying makeup, apply a primer (page 175) to smooth over wrinkles and pores and to create a gentle barrier between skin and other makeup.

2. *Use clean tools.* With rosacea, it is super important to have clean makeup and applicators to keep from further irritation. It is best to use brushes rather than sponges because sponges are more difficult to clean.

3. *Think dewy.* Use a gel or cream foundation (page 184) and concealer (page 178). These products are much more moisturizing than powder, which can settle in fine lines and on top of flakiness on the skin, making it seem more pronounced.

4. *Be easy on the eyes.* Many people with rosacea also experience symptoms in their eyes (redness, itchiness, gritty sensation), so it's best to use very mild products. Avoid liquid eyeliner and waterproof mascara. Liquid eyeliner tends to run and waterproof mascara is very difficult to remove without having to use chemical-based makeup remover.

acne-prone skin

Redheads can be more prone to acne because they have thinner skin. Many redheads, even those who have surpassed their teenage years, suffer from acne and/or breakouts.

"redhead friendly" tip: Stick to a simple skin regimen that helps control skin.

1. *Cleanser and lotion.* Before bed, wash your face with a cleanser that is free of harmful chemicals and works well with sensitive skin. Next, make sure to apply a lightweight lotion. Since a redhead's skin is typically sensitive and thin, make sure not to overwash your face! If you feel your skin does not need to be washed in the morning or night, simply splash lukewarm water on your face, dry and apply a lightweight lotion.

"redhead friendly" tip: When choosing a lotion for redheads, make sure the lotion is almost clear because it gives insight into what is going in your skin. If it's too heavy, it could be packed with more ingredients (sometimes an increase in chemicals) and could cause breakouts.

2. *Sleep.* It cures many acne problems because the skin is rejuvenated after those glorious eight hours of recommended rest.

3. *Acne scars.* Now, what happens when there is scarring from acne? Thankfully, there are many "redhead friendly" remedies and treatments that will help skin look refreshed in no time:

   a. The best thing you can do is choose a product or natural remedy that lightens the skin just a little bit, to allow the scarring to look not so pronounced. You can do this by selecting a foundation (liquid and/or powder) a shade lighter than your skin tone. Use your breastbone and neck color as a guide, since it's commonly the most natural shade on a woman.

b. If acne scars don't fade away on their own, it may be time to schedule an appointment with a dermatologist. Simple laser skin resurfacing can even out the skin surface and increase new collagen formation to help fill in acne scars. The fillers do need to be repeated every four to six months because the product reabsorbs into the skin over time, but it is totally worth it in the long run.

c. Redheads are stereotypically known to have the least amount of patience, but it does comes in hand in circumstances like this. If you have a new pimple and have a little bit of scarring, it may take a few months for the skin to repair.

d. Avoid foods with refined sugar as they will cause inflammation and redness and can make scars appear more visible.

e. The most important thing you can do when you have scarring is to apply sunscreen. The scarred area can be very sensitive to the sun and even worsen if it isn't protected.

"redhead friendly" tip: Use fresh lemon juice and apply to scars with a cotton ball. Allow it to sit for 15 minutes. The lemon works as a natural bleaching agent.

If you're more of a product kind of gal, try Clinique Even Better Clinical Dark Spot Corrector, which helps to reverse hyperpigmentation and prevent further discoloration. If you're suffering from puffy skin, try a cortisone cream to calm the skin first.

4. *Face mapping.* Have you ever heard of face mapping? If not, it can be the key for unlocking the mysteries behind your problematic skin. Face mapping is a type of skin analysis that explains why and how certain areas of the face are connected to other parts of the body. If you ask us, it's pretty amazing stuff. Why do you break out in some areas and not others? Each area reflects a different part of your internal health, so what exactly do pimples on certain areas mean? With this face map as a guide, you can address the underlying causes of blemishes and correctly determine how to prevent them from recurring.

Always make sure to consult your physician prior to any dietary change.

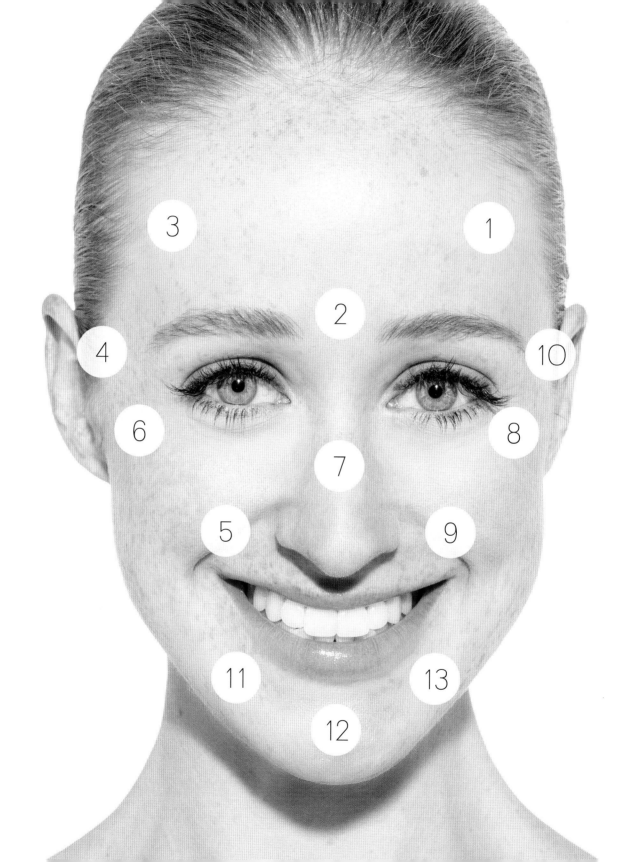

Areas 1 & 3: Bladder and Digestive System

Breaking out on your forehead may be a direct reflection of what's going on in your small intestine. High amounts of fat within your diet can lead you to break out across your forehead. Cleanse your diet with antioxidant-rich green tea and up your water intake to clear this area.

Area 2: Liver

If you break out near and/or the middle of your eyebrows, it is because you're stressing your liver. The liver breaks down fats, so you may be eating the wrong food. Alcohol and dairy are said to be the main causes for acne in this area. This is also an area that indicates food allergies. Consult your doctor for more information.

Areas 4, 6, 8 & 10: Kidneys

Spots close to your ear and even dark circles around the eyes can be caused by dehydration. Avoid salt and coffee.

Areas 5 & 9: Respiratory System

Those who smoke or have allergies tend to have acne here. But if you are breaking out a ¼ inch (6 mm) from the sides of your nose, this may reflect what's going on in your stomach. If you're constantly eating the wrong foods, not chewing thoroughly, eating too quickly or eating late at night, your skin may be breaking out as if to say, "Stop feeding my stomach this way!"

Area 7: Heart

Check your blood pressure and make sure you're not using makeup that irritates your sensitive redhead skin.

Area 12: Stomach

Consider a detox or adding more fiber to your diet to help with digestion.

Areas 11 & 13: Hormones

Stress and hormonal changes can sometimes be alleviated with more water and a few extra servings of dark, leafy greens. Additionally, breakouts in this area also indicate when you are ovulating.

mature skin

Redheads 35 and over may have visible attributes such as wrinkles, fine lines and sagging. Invest in products that have anti–aging components, such as moisturizers, serums and eye creams.

Since redheads are more sensitive to the sun and can frequently burn, they are at higher risk of wrinkles. This is why it's essential for redheads to introduce anti–aging treatments to their regimen early on.

Brown spots are a type of skin pigmentation problem that can be found with mature redheads, due to years of sun exposure and lack of sunscreen use. They appear flat; are tan, brown or black; and are commonly found on exposed skin such as the face, shoulders, hands and chest.

our "redhead friendly" favorite brands

$: Eucerin

$$: Lancome

$$$: Lamer

It is said that redheads bruise more easily, so redheads, take this advice next time you have a bruise: cover it up with a fragrance-free, hypoallergenic concealer with a yellow base, which will offset the blue discoloration.

"All redheads should also be aware of Light Therapy Treatments. They are amazing because they reduce inflammation, increase collagen production and make the skin super healthy. I love it for anyone with skin sensitivity because it makes the skin look perfect even after extraction."

—Joanna Vargas, founder of Joanna Vargas Skin Care in NYC

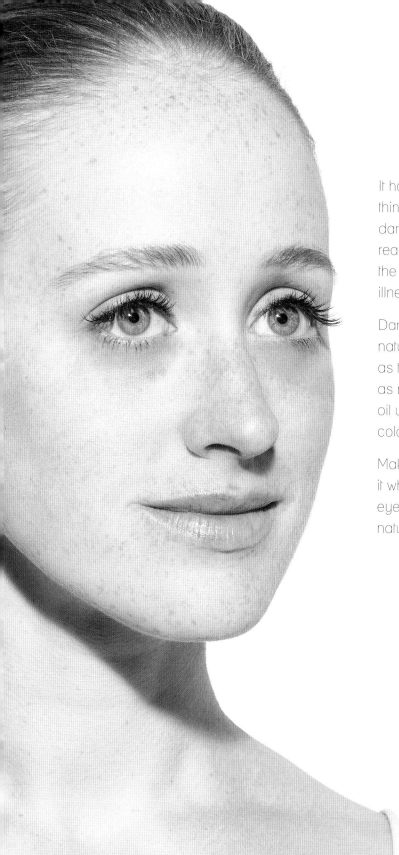

dark circles

It has been medically proven that redheads have thinner skin and that can result in skin issues like dark circles under the eyes. There are also several reasons that give rise to these ugly circles around the eyes, like lack of sleep, genetic factors, aging, illness and fatigue.

Dark circles can also be reduced with some natural methods, but you have to be very regular as the results are achieved gradually. Also, sleep as much as your body demands. Apply almond oil under the eye before going to bed and/or place cold tea bags on the eyes for some relaxation time.

Make concealer your best friend, but don't overdo it when applying. Apply a small amount around the eye and blend it properly with your fingers to give a natural and smooth look.

veins

It is very common for a redhead's veins to show, especially on the eyelid area. Apply a dime-size amount of concealer to both eyelids before applying your eye makeup. It will help get rid of any veins shining through.

back-of-arm bumps

Do you have small, rough red bumps around the hair follicles on the backs of your arms, legs and buttocks? If you touch the area, does it feel like chicken skin? Then your skin is probably experiencing *keratosis pilaris*. This is a very common skin condition seen in both kids and adults, especially those with sensitive skin. Most of the time, it develops during puberty, and can flare up with any extreme hot or cold. It can worsen during the cold winter months, when your skin is the most dry. Always make sure to moisturize these areas. If you see it developing in other areas and becoming more irritated, please consult a dermatologist.

These red patches are also a form of eczema. You will notice the bumps tend to get worse during the summer months because of the heat and humidity. Always apply sunscreen to the problem area, moisturize and cleanse with all-natural soaps. Seek a dermatologist if the condition worsens.

it's all about confidence!

Be strong and confident regardless if you have rosacea, acne, mature skin or if you're in the midst of a flare-up or notice another change in your skin. Spend some extra time on your hair and outfit so you feel confident.

makeup removal

Ever get the *don't-want-to-take-your-makeup-off* lazy syndrome? We get it all the time, especially after an entire day of work. Sleeping with your makeup on should be avoided at all times. It clogs pores and causes breakouts and wrinkles. It can also irritate the eyes, causing dryness, scratched cornea and blurred vision.

You have to give your redhead skin a break and let it breathe. So why not do it while you're sleeping? Take off makeup before cleansing, this will get the skin ready for a great cleanse. Make sure the makeup remover is non–oily and alcohol-free. This will avoid eye irritation.

Wear contacts? We advise taking them out before applying makeup remover to avoid eye irritation.

our "redhead friendly" favorites

Liquid Makeup Removers

$: Lumene Waterproof Eye Makeup Remover

$$: Clinique Rinse-Off Eye Makeup Solvent

Makeup Removal Wipes

$: Almay Oil-Free Makeup Remover Towelettes

$$: tarte Fresh Eyes Maracuja Waterproof Eye Makeup Remover Wipes

DIY

Coconut oil, jojoba oil and olive oil are three great oils for removing makeup.
Apply to a cotton swab to gently remove makeup.

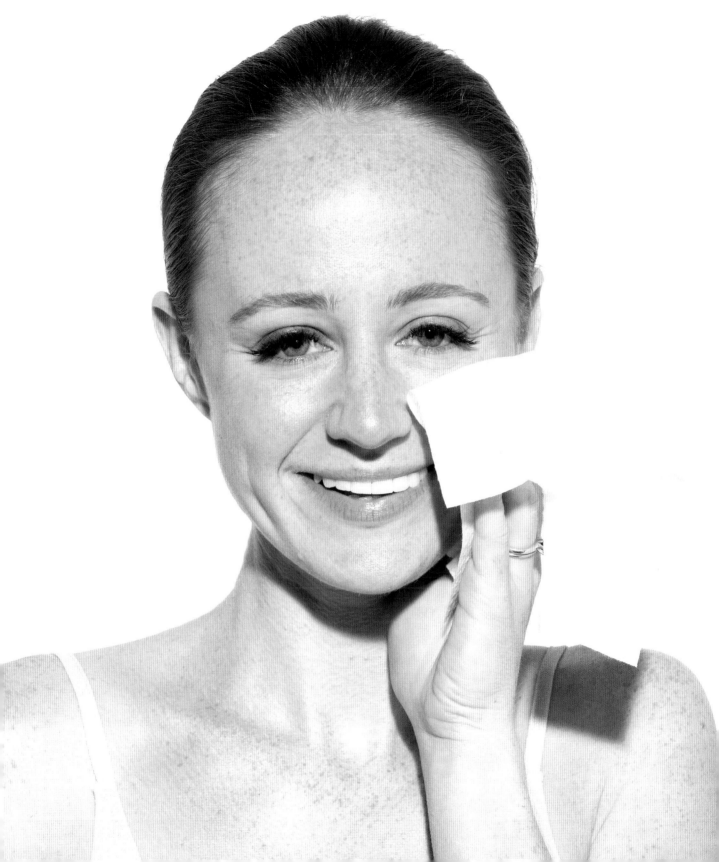

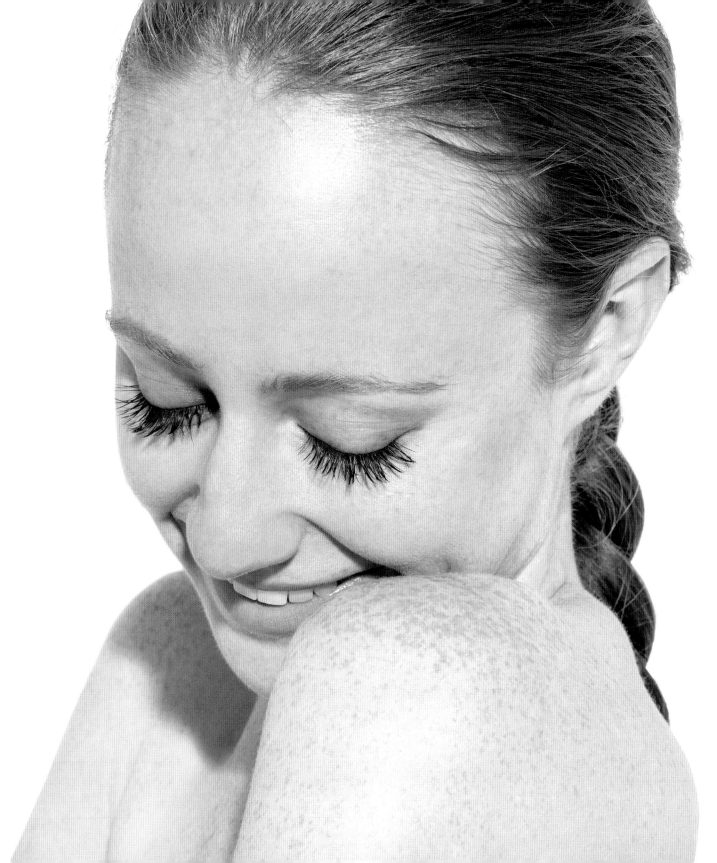

freckles:
the best accessory

Freckles are seasoning for your face. They make you spicy!

Freckles are tan and/or brownish spots that occur on sun-exposed skin.

I (Stephanie) went through an *I hate my freckles* stage and tried to cover them with heavy makeup. When I was younger, I recall reading *Freckle Juice* by Judy Blume and thinking, "I am Nicky." Nicky is a character in the book who had many freckles and wanted to get rid of them, while Nicky's classmate, Andrew, wanted to drink freckle juice because he so badly wanted to have freckles. At the time, I wanted my freckles gone, just like Nicky. Years later, I slowly learned more and more people are like Andrew, wishing they had freckles just like me! Freckles are a part of my everyday life and I could not imagine being a redhead without them.

"A redhead should get her freckles checked annually.
If you notice a growth that is growing rapidly, bleeds, changes color
or is asymmetrical, go see your dermatologist right away."

—Dr. Leslie Baumann, dermatologist and founder of
Baumann Cosmetic Dermatology in Miami

"I still have a difficult relationship with my freckles, as much as I hate to say it. When I was younger, I was teased for them—I vividly remember a friend taking pleasure in 'counting' them in front of a group on the playground— and then as you get older, you want to look older and more sophisticated, and freckles fight that idea. My top makeup tip for redheads with freckles: even if you're not in love with them, don't try to cover them with thick foundation—you'll look insane in photos. I know firsthand. When I was in high school and even well into my twenties, I tried so hard to obliterate my freckles with concealer, cream foundation and powder, that I ended up looking like I was 30 years older than I was. In my college graduation photo, I looked like Count Dracula. Look to Julianne Moore for inspiration: her freckles look more prominent in some photos, subtler in others, but she never 'blanks' them out completely."

—Jessica Matlin, deputy beauty editor at *Cosmopolitan* magazine

365 days of sunscreen

Redheads are more susceptible to melanoma. A mutation in a gene called MC1R gives redheads their hair color and fair skin, and now a new U.S. study suggests this same mutation triggers a cancer-causing signaling pathway when redheads are exposed to ultraviolet (UV) radiation. So, it's extremely important for redheads to wear sunscreen every single day.

SPF= sun protection factor

It refers to the ability of a sunscreen to block ultraviolet B rays (UVB), which cause sunburns, but not ultraviolet A rays (UVA), which are more closely linked to deeper skin damage. Both UVB and UVA contribute to the risk of skin cancer.

COTZ= contains only titanium and zinc

Titanium and zinc are important because they provide broad spectrum protection and use minerals that reflect UV rays, rather than chemicals that absorb UV rays.

"My top skincare product for every redhead is sunscreen."

—Joanna Vargas, founder of Joanna Vargas Skin Care in NYC

why higher SPFs aren't better
and why reapplying is everything

As a redhead, do you assume that SPF 100 will protect your fair skin better than SPF 30? SPF is not a consumer-friendly number. It is logical for someone to think that SPF 30 is twice as good as SPF 15 and so on. But that is not how it works.

An SPF 30 offers sunscreen protection for UVB light of 97%, an SPF 50 offers sunscreen protection of 98% for UVB light and an SPF 100 offers 99% protection for UVB light. You'll notice the differences in percentages are not that great, yet the numbers for SPF are.

The other problem with using high SPF values is that many people will not reapply their sunscreen. The recommendations are that you reapply sunscreen every two hours. The other problem is that many choose a high SPF, such as 70, that may not even block both UVA and UVB rays. It's essential for sunscreens to block both variations of rays to keep the skin protected.

The lesson here is to always use an SPF that protects against both UVA and UVB rays, and that using SPF 30 is doctor recommended. But make sure to reapply every 45 minutes to an hour to keep fair skin protected.

Many women, including redheads, are switching to coconut oil because of the chemicals in sunscreen. This a mistake! Redheads, oils and sun do not mix. Coconut oil will probably make the skin burn more. The very best skin protection is a physical blocker such as zinc oxide.

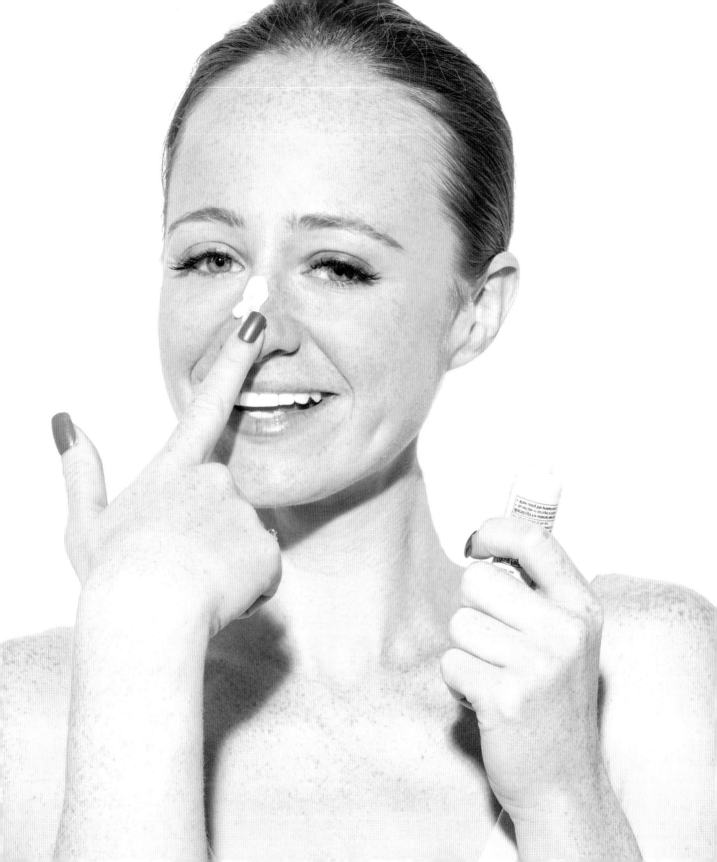

what to look for when choosing
a great sunscreen

Broad spectrum. Protects against UVA and UVB rays.

Water resistant. Lasts longer in the water.

All-natural ingredients. Free of toxins and chemical properties.

Sunscreen typically maintains its strength for about three years. After that time period, it is less effective. If your SPF doesn't have an expiration date, be sure to write on the bottle when the sunscreen was bought.

don't forget to put sunscreen
on these eight areas

1. Lips
2. Ears (especially the tops and backs of the ears)
3. Under the chin
4. Tops of feet and toes
5. Back of heels (along the tendons and bottoms of feet)
6. Hairline and scalp, regardless of hair type
7. Back of knees
8. Buttocks, if wearing a swimsuit

our "redhead friendly" favorites

stick

$: Neutrogena Ultra Sheer Face + Body Stick Sunscreen Broad Spectrum SPF 70

body lotion

$: Alba Botanica Very Emollient Mineral Sunscreen

$$: La Roche-Posay Anthelios 50 Mineral Tinted Ultra Light Sunscreen Fluid

face lotion

$$: Murad Oil Free Sunscreen Broad Spectrum SPF 30 PA+++

$$: MDSolarSciences Mineral Creme SPF 50 Broad Spectrum UVA-UVB

spray

$$: Sun Bum Sunscreen Spray SPF 15

wipes

$$: Supergoop! SPF 30 Sunscreen Swipes for Sensitive Skin

active

$$: COOLA Body SPF 15 Unscented Sunscreen Spray

baby

$$: California Baby Super Sensitive (No Fragrance)
Broad Spectrum SPF 30+ Sunscreen

to spray tan
or not to spray tan

When I (Adrienne) was a teenager, I hated my fair skin. Unlike Stephanie, who was full of gorgeous freckles, my skin was very light and I did what I thought was best: I piled on sunless tanner from head to toe. Granted, I never went the natural route and chose a dark tanner. It resulted in dark orange skin, which I proudly wore throughout high school and college. When I met my husband, he loved my light skin and convinced me to stop using the instant tanner. Now, I embrace my skin and know the shade I was born with looks best with my complexion.

There are occasions when both of us, Adrienne and Stephanie, will apply a gradual tanner. But we never go crazy. We've become so proud of our skin and love every bit of it. If you desperately want a tan, there are fantastic products on the market to give your redhead skin a beautiful glow.

what to avoid when faux tanning

Anything you put on your skin soaks right into the bloodstream. Like we recommend with all products, do your best to try all-natural sunless tanners and opt for shades one or two times darker than your natural skin tone.

five tips on how to prep skin for sunless tanners

1. Shave first, then exfoliate with an oil-free scrub. Extra oil can prevent sunless tanners from absorbing into the skin.

2. If you choose to wax, do it 24 hours in advance to avoid irritation.

3. Avoid moisturizing immediately before a sunless tanner is applied and refrain from using skin oils. The sunless tanning product will not properly absorb and could leave a streaky finish.

4. Visit your local beauty retail store and ask a skin specialist to demo and/or recommend sunless tanner products for your skin tone. Faux tanner comes in spray, lotion and mousse. The specialist can guide you in the right direction.

5. Make sure you have a full mirror handy so you can see your entire body when applying.

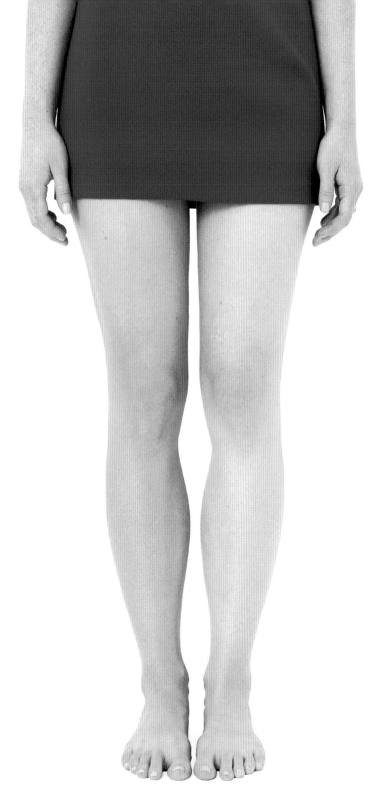

how to apply sunless tanner

Celebrity skin finishing and sunless tanning expert Fiona Locke shares her know-how on the best way to apply a sunless tanner.

1. Use a tanning mitt to get the perfect tan. This can be purchased at your local beauty store or online.

2. Start with the legs and work your way up in long, even strokes blending the product over each body part. First the legs, tummy, back, arms, chest and lastly, the face.

3. Blend the remaining product on the mitt evenly all over the face, sweeping down over the jaw and onto the neck. You can also apply a small amount of mousse to a makeup sponge and apply to face. It is always better to start with less and add more later once you know how your skin will take to the tan. Each individual skin tone will react differently.

4. The last areas of the body to tan are the hands and feet. Take the tanning mitt and swipe a light layer over the tops of the hands and feet. When the tanning application is complete, take a damp cloth and clean the nail beds and remove any product that may be on your palms.

after application

1. Wait at least 8 to 10 hours to shower, swim or work out because the product is still absorbing into skin and developing.

2. Use a rich body lotion to keep skin hydrated.

3. Avoid oil; it will break down your tan. Pat your skin dry after you shower, and when shaving legs use a little hair conditioner on the skin and very light pressure with a razor.

our "redhead friendly" favorites

$$: St. Tropez Self Tan Bronzing Mousse and Tan Application Mitt

$$: Vita Liberata pHenomenal Bronzing Mousse with Mitt

Tip: Want an immediate tan? Choose a product like Tan Towel's Illuma Glow Bronzing Body Lotion. It does not contain tanning agents but works as a temporary topical bronzer to add tint. Simply apply a small amount of product directly onto the skin and blend well in circular motions. Apply sparingly and distribute evenly.

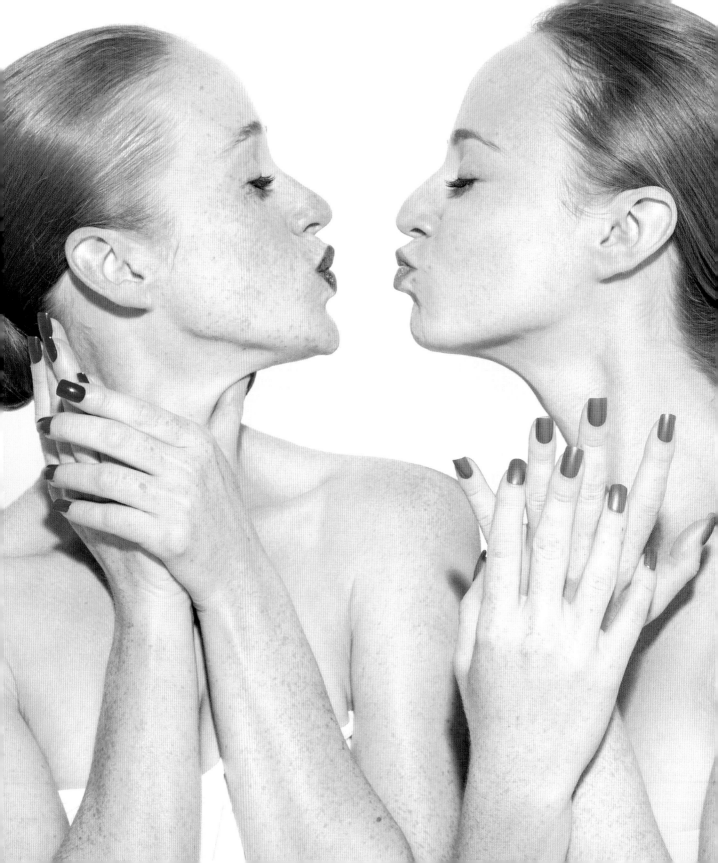

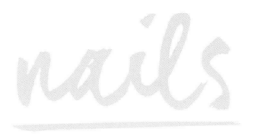

nails

Your red hair is looking flawless. Makeup is complete. Did you forget about your nails?

"Our nails naturally have a low oil and moisture content and therefore they can become dry and brittle. Hydration is crucial to our health in all facets, including our skin and nails! One of the biggest problems I see when working with clients and on-set is that women's nails, cuticles and hands are extremely dry. Topically, think of your nails and hands like your face. You wouldn't wash your face and not apply a moisturizer, but so often we wash our hands over and over and don't apply hand lotion. Keep a hand lotion that hydrates and protects your skin."

—Deborah Lippmann, celebrity manicurist

With so many redhead nail colors on the market, our number one advice is to choose a color that will express your redhead personality. There are no rules when it comes to wearing a certain color other than to *rock it*!

redheads can be described as

Mischievous • Temperamental • Feisty

Stubborn • Fiery • Confident

Go for a nail shape that suits you. A round, short nail is very classic and easy to maintain. A long, almond-shaped or oval nail elongates your fingers and makes your nails pop.

Redheads have sensitive skin, especially around the cuticle area. It is very important to treat the cuticle like you would any other part of the skin.

how to properly treat cuticles

1. Soak the hands in warm water for 2 to 3 minutes.

2. Apply an exfoliating cuticle treatment, massage into the cuticles and push back gently.

3. Since redheads have sensitive skin, the cuticles can be very sensitive. Instead of cutting the cuticles, push them back. It's much healthier. Make sure to clarify this to your nail technician at your next appointment.

4. Moisturize the cuticle, nail bed and hands regularly.

"Cuticles are important because they act as a barrier to keep bacteria at bay and should only be pushed back, never cut. Cutting them can potentially lead to irritation and infection, which can result in permanent damage to the nail or worse."

—Deborah Lippmann, celebrity manicurist

ten ways to get healthy nails

1. *Don't bite your nails.* This will make nails look unkempt and it's very unsanitary.

2. *Avoid gel manicures.* Over time, they leave nails soft, dull and damaged. Plus redheads should always stay away from UV lights, which are part of the application process. The lighting is incredibly damaging to the skin.

3. *Use cuticle oil.* This will hydrate the cuticle area.

4. *Color, color, breathe.* Color, color and breathe. It's important to give your nails a color break.

5. *Scrubs.* Moisturize hands by washing and exfoliating with scrubs.

6. *Hand lotions.* Moisturize hands by applying hand lotion daily.

7. *Maintain a healthy lifestyle.* Nails say a lot about your health. Look out for unhealthy signs such as white and ridged nail beds.

8. *Never push down cuticles when dry.* You want them to be wet or else they will become irritated.

9. *Go to a trusted nail salon.* Your nails are part of your body, so make sure you're going to a sanitary salon.

10. *Let your nails define you!*

deborah lippmann's red-carpet-ready nails

The ease of manicuring all comes down to a well-groomed nail. A professional red-carpet-ready manicure is executed simply by following the easy steps outlined in the Five Step Manicure:

Step 1. *Cleanse.* Saturate a piece of cotton with nail polish remover.

Step 2. *Shape.* Shape the nail so it mirrors the cuticle and elongates the fingers. Remember to use gentle motions to prevent breakage.

Step 3. *Exfoliate.* To prepare nails for lacquer or to create a beautiful buff, use a 4-way nail buffer. This all-in-one exfoliator offers four unique fabrics to make grooming as easy as one, two, three. Side one works to smooth away dullness, side two buffs away ridges and side three smoothens the nail. Stop here if you are prepping for your polish, but if opting for a natural buffed look, finish with side 4 to reveal an unbelievable shine.

Step 4. *Treat.* One of the most important steps. Treatment softens and hydrates the nails and cuticles. Gently push back cuticles as described above and apply oil onto the base of each nail.

Step 5. *Finish.* Cleanse away any oil, dirt or residue from the nail plate with gentle soap and water. Once dry, apply your favorite base coat, per your nail concerns, two layers of nail polish and finally the top coat to finish it off.

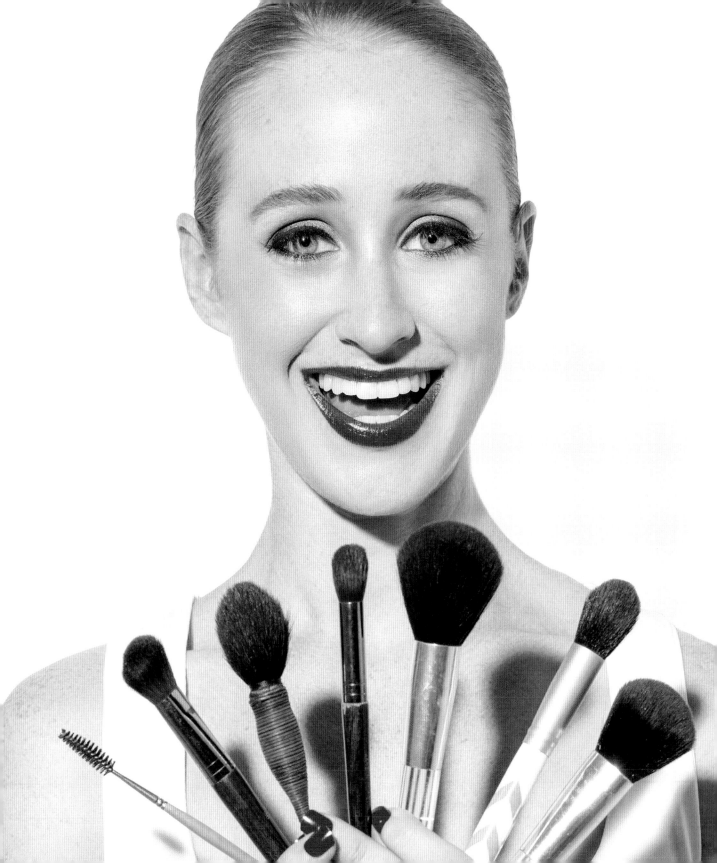

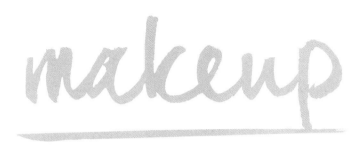

makeup

I can sum up our high school dance makeup in one word: disaster. Like most teenagers, you head to the mall or department store to get your makeup done. We, along with our blonde and brunette friends, would look to our local makeup artists for that glamorous look. But in our case, it consisted of foundation that was too dark, eye makeup that made us look like raccoons and eyebrows that matched the color of our hair (something you should never do).

It was an ugly situation!

During my junior year of high school, I (Stephanie) had a bad experience with my makeup artist, and Adrienne had to meet me in the mall bathroom, where she helped me wash off the makeup and we enhanced my look in a subtle, natural way.

I am sure some of you have had far worse happen to you, and some of you luckily found great makeup artists. Always call a store before you make an appointment and ask if anyone has worked on redheads before. If they sound confident, chances are they'll nail your makeup.

Because of this so-called struggle, Adrienne and I had to learn *How to be a Redhead* and do our makeup ourselves. Over the years, we have found the perfect makeup products for those with red hair.

makeup tools

①

sponge

A makeup applicator used to blend and apply liquid foundation.

"redhead friendly" tip: Before applying liquid foundation to the sponge, lightly wet it with water. This will create a natural, dewy look. Next, dab the sponge over the skin, working on blending all throughout.

our "redhead friendly" favorite

$$: beautyblender original

②

eyelash curler

A makeup tool that curls your lashes.

"redhead friendly" tip: Use an eyelash curler before mascara or else your mascara will get ruined, making your lashes stick together. Always start at the inner corner of your eye, working your way out. Make sure the curler is as close to the root as possible, hold for a few seconds, let go and repeat.

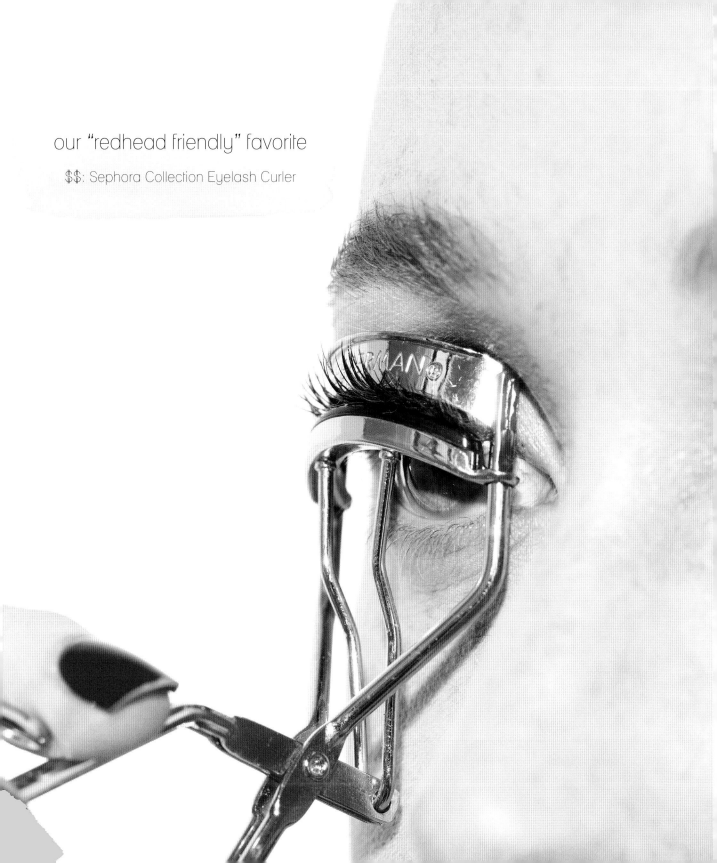

our "redhead friendly" favorite

$$: Sephora Collection Eyelash Curler

pencil sharpener

A handheld device for creating a point on a pencil.

"redhead friendly" tip: We recommend dual-blade sharpeners. That way, no matter the size of your eyeliner (skinny or wide), it will sharpen beautifully.

our "redhead friendly" favorite

$: Make Up For Ever Double Barrel Pencil Sharpener

eyebrow tweezer

A handheld tool for removing eyebrow and facial hair.

"redhead friendly" tip: Always have a pair of tweezers in your makeup bag and remember to tweeze one hair at a time in the direction of hair growth. This will avoid the hair being aggravated and allow for smooth hair removal.

our "redhead friendly" favorite

$$: Tweezerman

makeup mirror

A stand-alone or handheld tool used to see your reflection.

"redhead friendly" tip: Owning a stand-alone and compact mirror will make your makeup application so much easier. Always make sure you are applying makeup in natural light.

magnifying mirror

Great for up close and personal makeup and beauty tasks such as tweezing or applying eyeliner.

compact mirror

Great for traveling and needing a makeup retouch, especially on your lips.

"You cannot achieve good makeup without good tools."

— François Nars, makeup artist and founder of NARS Cosmetics

Makeup brushes are a must. They are the most sanitary way to apply makeup and make almost every look flawless. Well-made brushes will make your makeup look best, letting your face breathe without looking cakey. Your face is a canvas, so treat it like one!

foundation brush

There are two kinds of foundation brushes:

flat brush

Perfect for a light, flawless application.

stippling brush

Perfect for a more airbrushed look.

eye shadow brush

Perfect for blending and big enough to add a pop of color to your eyelids.

eyeliner brush

An angled brush that is perfect for getting right to the root in order to tackle those blonde lashes.

4

powder brush

A very common brush used to apply powder foundation.

5

eyebrow brush

Most redheads have very light eyebrows, and a great angled brush can perfect those arches and fill in every hair.

6

concealer brush

Firm enough to conceal and hide your dark circles and blemishes.

7

blending blush brush

This particular brush gives you the ability to dab your blush in a dotted rhythmic motion, causing a more blended effect. That's right—do not sweep brush across cheekbones.

8

bronzer brush

A short, stocky brush that is great for blending bronzer.

lip brush

We love a lip brush for many reasons. It creates an easy application, gives you more control and the ability to blend colors.

lash and brow comb

Great tool to use before doing anything with your eyebrows. It lifts the hair up and gets any clumps or straggly hairs out.

Cleaning makeup brushes is very similar to cleaning hairbrushes (page 55). Simply use baby shampoo to thoroughly cleanse the brush, rinse and lay flat down on a towel to dry overnight.

our "redhead friendly" favorite brands

$$: MAC Cosmetics

$$: Clinique

makeup base

Our makeup steps include: prepping skin, primer, concealer, foundation, eye makeup, eyebrows, bronzer/blush and lipstick. We call this process: *GlamouRED*. Follow us as we show you, step by step, which products will work best for you and how to apply them.

step 1. prep skin (using tips on pages 119–129.)

step 2. primer

After prepping the skin, it's time to apply primer. We always call primer the "the stepchild of makeup" because many people think it's optional or do not know it exists. It is a must! Primer helps makeup last longer, while creating a base for concealer and foundation. We suggest a lightweight primer that will not weigh skin down.

our "redhead friendly" favorites

$: Rimmel London Lasting Finish Primer

$$: Cover FX Mattifying Primer with Anti-Acne Treatment

"For redheads, a yellow or green primer is great for counteracting redness."

—Lauren Gott, redhead makeup artist

how to apply

1. Apply a dime-size amount to the top of the hand. Think of this area of the hand as a painting palette.

2. Take a makeup sponge or use your finger to apply a few dime-size amounts of primer between your thumb and index finger. Fingers give you a more natural, fresh look because the heat of your hands warms and thins the makeup. For more coverage, use a brush.

3. Begin applying the primer on the forehead and work downward toward the chin.

4. When more primer is needed, return to the hand palette for more. If you have wrinkles, primer works beautifully because it fills in those areas.

knowing what color primer to use on the skin can be very challenging. here's an easy breakdown:

Clear. The most common color. Great for smoothing the skin.

Yellow or green. We are huge fans of these two colored primers.

Pink. This color brightens a redhead's complexion.

"For redheads so pale the skin lacks vibrancy, a pink primer would liven the skin. I've never used purple primer on a redhead. Purple is generally used to awaken sallow, yellow skin, which is uncommon among redheads."

—Lauren Gott, redhead makeup artist

other "redhead friendly" must-have primers

lash primer

Preps the lashes before applying mascara.

Our Favorite: It Cosmetics Tightline Mascara Primer

eye shadow primer

Creates a base for the eye shadow by preventing creasing to make
the eye makeup pop all day.

Our Favorite: Urban Decay Eyeshadow Primer Potion

lip primer

Adds moisture before applying color to the lips.

Our Favorite: Too Faced Lip Insurance Lip Primer

Tip #1: Primer will not cover up freckles and a little goes a very long way.

Tip #2: Always apply makeup in natural lighting because it is the purest light
and will make sure you do not miss anything.

step 3. concealer

Stephanie's must-have beauty product is concealer because she has very dark circles and puffy eyes, especially during allergy season. This product is great for any redhead, especially those who have veins on their eyelids and underneath their eyes. Concealer quickly hides dark spots too.

how to apply

1. Apply by drawing a small triangle underneath each eye. This will actually lift the face and avoid raccoon eyes.

Tip #1: Use concealer on the eyelids in replacement of an eye shadow primer. Simply apply it to a clean face before applying eye shadow.

Tip #2: For blue-toned under-eye circles (very common in redheads), use a peach concealer to brighten the eyes.

different types of concealers

1

stick

Concealer in a stick form is great for targeting specific areas on the skin, and it's ideal for those looking for medium to full coverage. With a stick concealer, you have the ability to control where the product is going, which is great for those redheads not looking to cover up their freckles. Make sure to always dot and blend.

our "redhead friendly" favorites

$: Maybelline Concealer

$$: NUDESTIX Concealer Pencil

2

cream

Concealer packaged in a circular container or palette. Since cream concealers tend to have a thick, pasty consistency, they are great for achieving full coverage. We do not recommend this product for a redhead who enjoys showcasing her freckles, since the texture tends to conceal everything where it is applied.

our "redhead friendly" favorites

$$: Benefit Cosmetics Boi-ing Concealer

3

liquid

Concealer packaged in liquid form is great for all types of coverage. You can apply with a clean finger and concealer brush by making dots where you want the concealer to go with your finger and gently blending with a concealer brush. A little goes a long way.

our "redhead friendly" favorites

$: L.A. Girl HD PRO Conceal

$$: Tarte Cosmetics Maracuja Creaseless Concealer

4

powder

Concealer packaged in powder form is great for light coverage, especially when looking to conceal a blemish or scar.

our "redhead friendly" favorites

$: e.l.f. Cosmetics Mineral Concealer

$$: bareMinerals

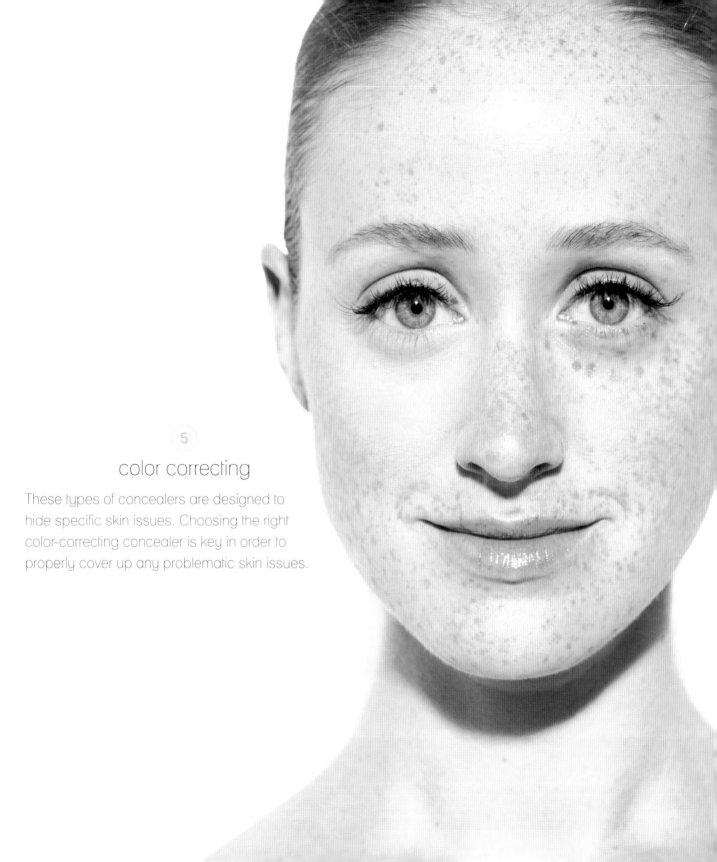

5

color correcting

These types of concealers are designed to hide specific skin issues. Choosing the right color-correcting concealer is key in order to properly cover up any problematic skin issues.

yellow

Best for counteracting scarring, bruises and acne blemishes.

green

Best for getting rid of redness.

peach/orange

Best for blue-toned under-eye circles.

purple/lavender

Best to cancel out yellow undertones.

blue

Best for those who have an orange tint to their skin.

tip #3: Apply concealer right before foundation. After applying the *GlamouRED* process, go in and apply a few dots of concealer to any areas missed or to any eye shadow, eyeliner or mascara residue that may be on the skin.

tip #4: Apply concealer to lips before applying lipstick, focusing on the middle section of the pout. This will make the lips look fuller!

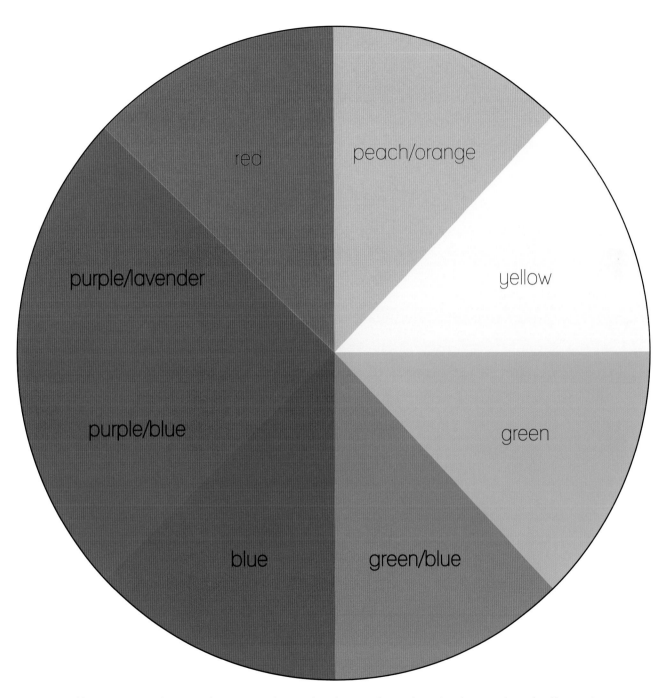

red

peach/orange

purple/lavender

yellow

purple/blue

green

blue

green/blue

Always remember—colors opposite each other on the color wheel cancel each other out.

step 4. how to find the perfect foundation— a redhead's dream come true

Has this situation happened to you?

A beautiful redhead is at the cosmetic counter at a department store and is searching tirelessly for the foundation that will perfectly match her complexion. A makeup artist, dressed in a white lab coat, approaches her and asks, "I'd be happy to help you choose a foundation. Are you a warm toned or a cool toned?"

The redhead looks at her blankly and says, "I'm not sure."

Of course, the makeup artist can look at a redhead's skin and decipher if the skin is cool or warm toned, but it's also important for a redhead to know about her skin inside and out. So, if she's faced with deciding herself, she'll be able to choose the perfect shade.

When Adrienne was in high school, she struggled with accepting her fair skin and would use a dark tan shade for foundation. She figured it would mask her light skin and make her look like everyone else. Unfortunately she had a dark, unblended makeup line on her chin for most of her teens until she discovered the foundation shade that made her skin glow.

"PALE? I'm not pale. It's called porcelain and I'm rockin' it."

"I smooth foundation down the front of the neck to 'warm it up' to blend flawlessly with the jawline/face."

—Brett Freedman, makeup artist and owner/creator of Brett Freedman Beauty

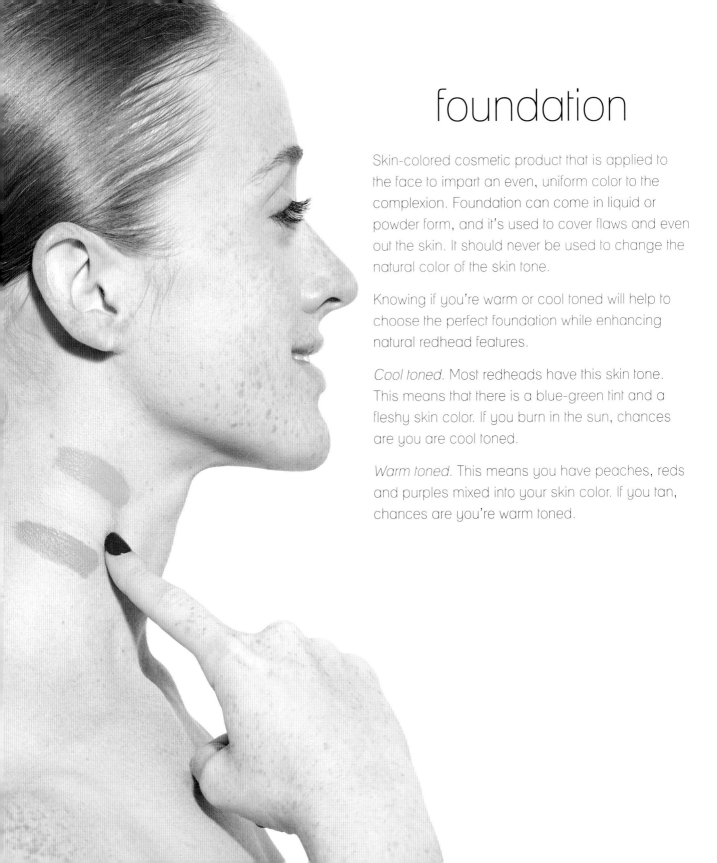

foundation

Skin-colored cosmetic product that is applied to the face to impart an even, uniform color to the complexion. Foundation can come in liquid or powder form, and it's used to cover flaws and even out the skin. It should never be used to change the natural color of the skin tone.

Knowing if you're warm or cool toned will help to choose the perfect foundation while enhancing natural redhead features.

Cool toned. Most redheads have this skin tone. This means that there is a blue-green tint and a fleshy skin color. If you burn in the sun, chances are you are cool toned.

Warm toned. This means you have peaches, reds and purples mixed into your skin color. If you tan, chances are you're warm toned.

Here's a simple quiz to find out if you're cool or warm toned:

1 Look at the inside of your wrists. What color do your veins predominantly appear?

a. More blue.
b. More green.

2 Try on a bright yellow or bright orange T-shirt. How do you look?

a. Washed out.
b. Beautiful. It gives me a glow!

3 After cleansing your face, put a piece of bright white paper next to your skin. How do you look?

a. Let me put it this way, I do not look my best.
b. Terrific! White is my color for sure.

4 What happens to your skin when you're out in the sun for a long time without sunscreen?

a. I burn instantly.
b. I might burn at first, but then I tan. I hardly ever sunburn.

5 Which group does your eye color fall under?

a. Golden brown, green, blue or hazel with gold flecks.
b. Black, deep brown, gray or hazel with deep-colored flecks.

If you answered more A, you are cool toned. If you answered more B, you are warm toned.

This simple answer will help you discover not only the best makeup, but the most complementary fashion items and the best shade of red hair if/when you ever need to dye or enhance your locks. This is the token to finding the perfect colors in your redhead life.

different types of foundation

Makeup with sunscreen is not enough to protect the skin. Always make sure to use sunscreen, even if your foundation has SPF in it.

(1)

loose powder

A mineral-based foundation.

how to apply

This is our favorite type of foundation for redheads because it is light and effortless.

1. Add a small amount of mineral powder to the lid of the product.

2. Swirl powder brush in the lid and tap away any excess off the brush—this will eliminate heavy, uneven application.

3. Apply in circular motions throughout.

our "redhead friendly" favorites

$: Physicians Formula Mineral Wear

$$: Laura Mercier Mineral Powder

Tip #1: Many loose powders have a gray undertone, which can make a redhead's skin look dull. Choose one with a cream undertone.

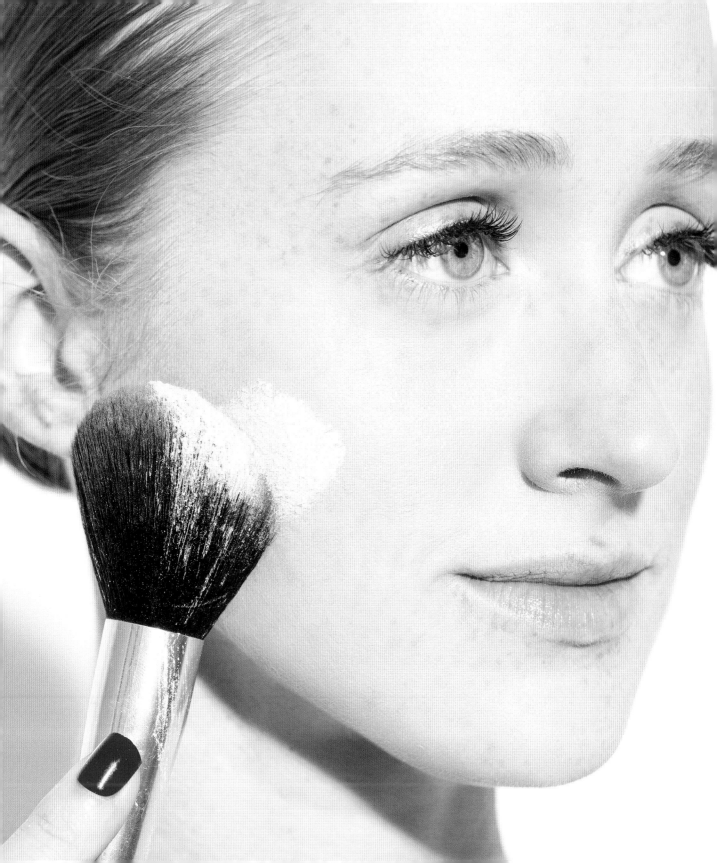

setting powder

Tip #1: Do not confuse traditional loose powder with setting powder. Setting powder helps to lock in the look, *not* perfect the skin. Setting powder is the secret to taking beautiful photos (and selfies).

our "redhead friendly" favorites

$$: Make Up For Ever HD Microfinish Powder

"Red hair is beautiful. It makes people happy. People smile and say hello to people with red hair. It's really quite extraordinary. I love the way red hair photographs in different lights. How it looks different at night. It's just so special."

—Margaret Nagle, screenwriter and producer

liquid

A liquid-based foundation.

how to apply

1. *For a sheer daytime look*, apply foundation with either the fingers or a makeup sponge.

2. *For a heavier evening look*, apply foundation using a foundation brush.

3. *For a dewy look*, dampen your sponge before applying foundation to it.

Tip #1: Foundation can be heavy. No one wants a foundation line around the jaw and chin. Make sure to *blend, blend, blend!* You want the neck and face to look the same shade. Lock it all in with a loose setting powder. This will blend the foundation even more.

our "redhead friendly" favorites

$: Almay Clear Complexion Blemish Healing Liquid Makeup

$$: Dermablend Smooth Liquid Camo Foundation

pressed

A compact and portable foundation. It applies lighter than a liquid foundation but heavier than loose powder.

how to apply

1. Begin with the spots you want to perfect and/or hide, including any redness or shine. For most women, it is under the eyes, the cheeks and the nose.

our "redhead friendly" favorites

$: Neutrogena Mineral Sheers Powder Foundation

$$: Clinique Almost Powder Makeup Broad Spectrum SPF 15

stick

A portable stick foundation. It applies similarly to a liquid foundation.

how to apply

1. Sticks tend to be heavy. We always advise redheads to lightly apply to *only* the areas that need it: uneven skin spots, blemishes and dark areas.

2. Dot the stick on these areas and lightly rub in with clean fingers or use a foundation brush/ sponge.

our "redhead friendly" favorite

$: e.l.f. Studio Moisturizing Foundation Stick

"Many foundations have SPF in them. It only has enough protection for everyday use if it contains broad spectrum SPF 30+ sunscreen."

—Dr. Robert J. Friedman, clinical professor at NYU School of Medicine, Department of Dermatology

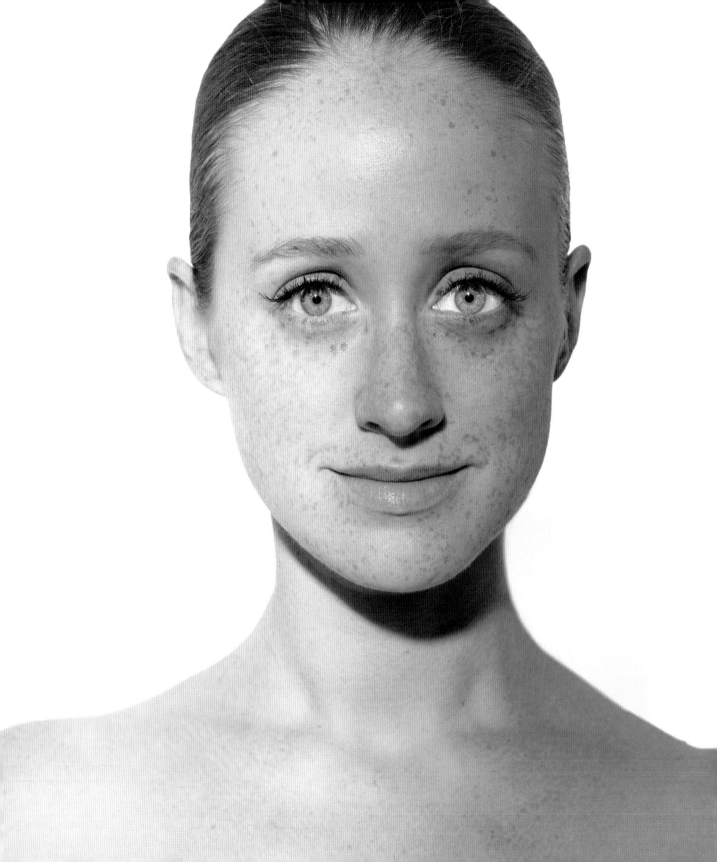

tricks for summer and winter

1. In the summer, keep foundation sheer with a tinted moisturizer in a slightly warmer shade to emphasize the color of gorgeous redhead skin (and freckles, if you have them).

2. In the winter months, emphasize the underlying skin tone color and use thicker moisturizer and foundation. You can cancel out redness with a yellow-based foundation and concealer.

other "redhead friendly" foundation-like products

(1)

BB cream

BB stands for *beauty balm* or *blemish balm*. This type of cream was created by dermatologists for patients who had gone through laser skin surgery. It reduces oils, minimizes pores and hydrates skin. It can be worn by itself or with foundation, depending on if you are going for a light or heavy look. For extra protection, we always choose a cream that contains SPF.

our "redhead friendly" favorites

$: Garnier BB Cream

$$: Smashbox Camera Ready BB Cream

CC cream

CC stands for *color correcting*. This particular cream is made to adjust redness, which is very common in a redhead's skin.

our "redhead friendly" favorites

$: Almay Smart Shade CC Cream Complexion Corrector

$$: Cover FX CC Cream Time Release Tinted Treatment SPF 30

DD cream

DD stands for *dynamic duo*. Think of this particular cream as a BB cream and a CC cream in one. It controls blemishes, hydrates, protects, conceals and acts as a primer to the skin.

how to apply

For BB, CC and DD creams

1. Apply sunscreen to face.

2. Apply a dime-size amount of cream on top of the palm.

3. Use finger to gently blend the cream in a circular motion over the skin, focusing on problematic areas.

4. Depending on how much coverage you are looking for, you can continue with concealer and foundation. If you want freckles to shine, opt out of applying foundation.

tinted moisturizer

Looking for a moisturizer with a little kick? Tinted moisturizer is it! It's a perfect blend of skincare and makeup that hydrates skin and softens fine lines with a sheer hint of color for a healthy, dewy glow. We love rockin' this product on our skin during the summer months because it's light and non–oily. Opt for this product if you are looking for a moisturizer and foundation in one.

how to apply

1. After cleansing, apply a quarter-size amount to the face using the index finger (for a lighter look) or sponge/foundation brush (for a heavier look).

2. Do not use foundation after tinted moisturizer because it will feel and look heavy and unnatural. Bronzer and blush may be applied after.

Tip #1: Apply a dime-size amount of foundation to the palm of the hand, then apply a few drops of moisturizer to the foundation. Mix and apply to face. This will act as a tinted moisturizer without breaking the bank.

our "redhead friendly" favorite

$$: Laura Mercier Tinted Moisturizer

"Fair-skinned redheads with few to no freckles, or color elsewhere, can match their skin tone by applying to the jaw line. These redheads tend to be porcelain pink (choose a pale yellow tone, yellow or green primer to cancel natural redness) or translucent in skin tone. Freckled or slightly tanned redheads should consider their body color to match their face. I like picking a shade or two lighter than the darkest freckles. This appears the most natural and allows the freckles to peek through. Don't forget to apply a bit of sunscreen and foundation to the chest, which is so often overlooked by redheads and, as a result, red and/or sun damaged."

—Lauren Gott, redhead makeup artist

freckle-friendly foundation

"A face without freckles is like a night without stars."

If you have freckles, this section is dedicated to you!

The best types of foundations for freckled redheads are lightweight liquid foundations, mineral powders and/or tinted moisturizers that contain SPF.

how to apply

Whether applying liquid foundation or mineral powder, apply it only where you need coverage.

Tip #1: Stay away from heavy liquid foundations because they will actually cover up freckles. No one wants that!

Tip #2: Want freckles to pop? After applying foundation, dip a cotton swab in water and gently dot on face to expose freckles.

bronzer and blush

A pink-based blush and a subtle bronzer can make freckles glisten and pop. Simply sweep cheekbones with a pink blush and add a tiny bit of bronzer over the blush.

Tip #3: Stay away from products that are too glittery because it will take away from your beautiful angel kisses.

7

draw more on

Yes! You can draw more freckles on the skin and it's so easy to do.

how to apply

1. For a more natural look, opt for an eye pencil. Choose a color that is closest to the color of the freckles, whether it be dark blonde, red or brown.

2. Lightly dot the eye pencil on the skin, especially where the sun hits the face (along the cheekbone and under the eyes).

our "redhead friendly" favorite

: Topshop Freckle Pencil in Forever Young

step 5.
easy contouring

Can redheads contour and highlight?
The answer is yes! Contouring is the
art of bringing out the best features on
one's face, while adding definition to the
face. It is the illusion of perfectly chiseled
cheekbones and a very strong jawline.
The main trick for a redhead wanting
to achieve this look is knowing exactly
where to apply the correct bronzer and
highlighter, making sure not to cover up
freckles.

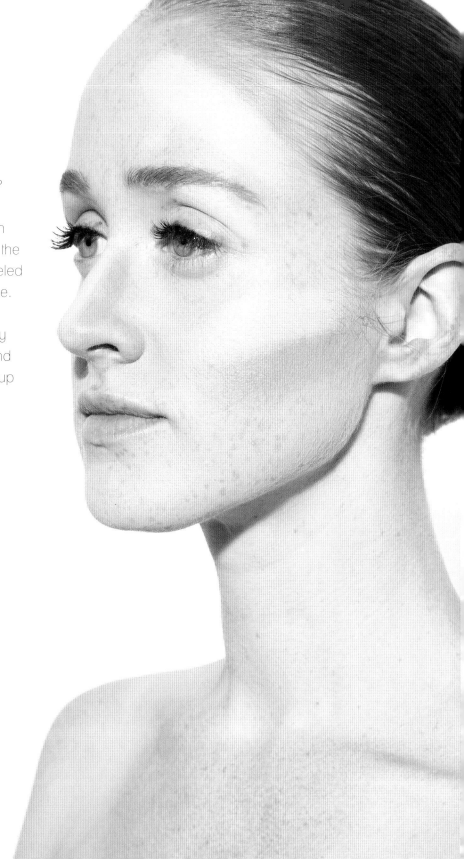

how to contour

1. Apply foundation (pages 188–192).

2. Choose a contour shade that is a few shades darker than your natural skin tone. This will be applied to places such as under the cheeks, sides of nose, jaw and temples.

3. Choose a highlighter shade that is a few shades lighter than your natural skin tone. This will be applied to the tops of the cheeks, brow bone area and under the eyes.

4. To bring out your cheekbones, apply the contour shade at the hollow part of the cheeks. Find this area by placing fingers on the side of the face. Feel that dip? Apply the shade right above the dip.

5. Contour a wide forehead by applying the darker contour shade to each temple and blend. To minimize a double chin, contour the chin by applying the darker contour shade along the jawline and blend down toward the neck.

6. Apply the highlighter shade under the eyes, on the brow bone and on the tops of the cheeks.

7. Take the makeup sponge and blend the contour shade and highlighter shade into the foundation. Blend in a circular motion to buff into the skin.

8. Set with translucent powder.

"The nose can be slimmed if applied on each side and highlighted on the bridge. A long nose can be truncated if applied at the tip of the nose. The only way to make contouring appear natural is by blending until you see no distinct lines."

—Lauren Gott, redhead makeup artist

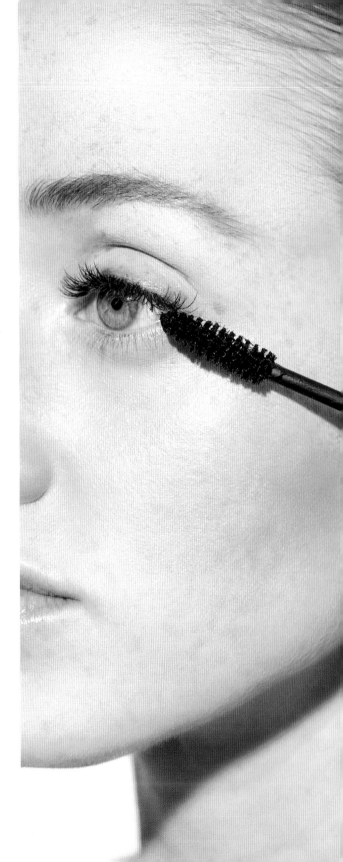

step 6. enhancing your red hair with eye makeup

In most instances, redheads have very fair eyelashes. It's important to define the eye with mascara, whether it is light brown, dark brown or jet black. Some feel completely comfortable rockin' their natural lashes with pure confidence (go for it!) but mascara gives the eye unbelievable definition. It even makes the hair pop MORE.

Our redheaded grandmother gave us our first mascara, which was Maybelline Great Lash in black. For that reason, we have a very strong love for black mascara. It's our go-to eye makeup product and, like most redheads, we can never leave the house without a few coats applied to each eye.

our "redhead friendly" favorites

$: Rimmel London ScandalEyes RetroGlam Extra Black

$: CoverGirl LashBlast Volume Mascara

$$: Tarte Cosmetics Lights, Camera, Lashes 4-in-1 Mascara

favorite mascara tips for redheads

1. *Black and brown combo.* Since many think red hair and black mascara looks too harsh, a great tip is to wear black on the top lashes and brown on the bottom. Keep makeup glamorous-looking and not overpowering by sticking with darker mascara, but keeping it lighter with eyeliner and eye shadow. It's most important that your makeup reflects your personality. If you love a bold eyeliner with deep mascara, have fun with it! If you're more conservative, stick with brown mascara and a nude eye shadow.

2. *Colored mascara.* If you love to experiment, rock brown, purple, blue, green and auburn mascara. Let your hair and colored mascara do the talking and keep the other makeup to a minimum.

3. *Hypoallergenic.* Do you suffer from itchy, dry, watery eyes? Try a hypoallergenic mascara. This means the product is free of allergens and is less likely to cause a reaction in people with allergies or sensitivities.

our "redhead friendly" favorites

$: Almay One Coat Thickening Mascara

$$: Physicians Formula Organic Wear 100% Natural Origin Mascara

4. *Avoid Waterproof.* For redheads with sensitive skin, we always recommend avoiding waterproof mascara. It is hard to remove and can create irritation around and in the eyes. Choose a mascara that easily comes off with cleanser and/or oils.

"It's all about the eyes. Redheads usually have fair lashes and brows. Black mascara does wonders in making a redhead's eyes pop instead of disappearing."

—Christiane Seidel, actress

how to conquer fair eyelashes

Step 1. Apply mascara from underneath and brush upward.

Step 2. If you feel like you can still see traces of blonde at the base of your eyelashes, wiggle the application wand at the base, then brush outward from underneath. It will cover up any blonde and make lashes look longer and thicker.

Step 3. Apply mascara on the other eye.

tips

+ If you happen to get mascara on the eyelid, take a wet cotton swab and remove the excess.

+ Use petroleum jelly to lengthen and moisturize the lashes.

+ If any fair lashes are showing through after applying mascara, cover them at the root with eyeliner.

+ If you have trouble applying mascara to bottom lashes, there are mascara products on the market that have tiny wands. Our "redhead friendly" favorite: NYX Cosmetics The Skinny Mascara.

eye shadow

A colored cosmetic product, typically in powder form, applied to the eyelids or around the eyes to accentuate them. Eye shadow can make the eyes and hair pop for redheads with either light or dark eyes. Depending on the color that complements you, eye shadows give a natural and glamorized look.

best eye shadow shades for different eye colors

green

A common eye color among redheads.

Best Colors: brown, nude, violet

blue

It is a naturally cool tone, so warmer shades tend to set this color on fire.

Best Colors: gray-brown, slate, eggplant

Tip #1: You always want to go with the opposite color on the color wheel. So if your eyes are warm toned, the best eye shadow shades are cool toned. If your eyes are cool toned, the best eye shadow shades are warm toned.

Red hair and blue eyes is the rarest combination in the world.

hazel

Hazel eyes contain a range of tones. They're somewhere in between green and brown and often have flecks of gold and gray. Because of their innate spectrum of colors, play up certain aspects of hazel eyes to transform the eye from boring to fabulous.

Best Colors: lavender, violet or plum

brown

Redheads with this color eye have the most options because mostly every eye shadow looks complementary.

Best Colors: warm bronze, purple, teal

how to apply

We call this easy four-step process *The Fiery Eye*.

1. Grab a paper towel and fold it into a square. Place the towel square underneath the eye, making sure the top is underneath the bottom lashes. This will prevent eye shadow residue from falling down the face.

2. Apply eye shadow primer to the lids (page 177). This will hold the shadow in place and eliminate creases.

3. Grab an eye shadow palette and eye shadow brush. Swirl the brush into the palette and apply on the lids.

4. If using multiple shades, always apply the dark color on the lower lid to keep the look polished. Keep lighter shadows on the top of the lid near the eyebrow.

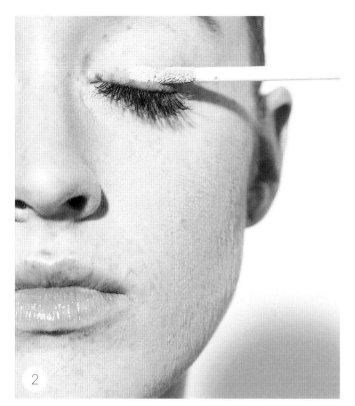

2

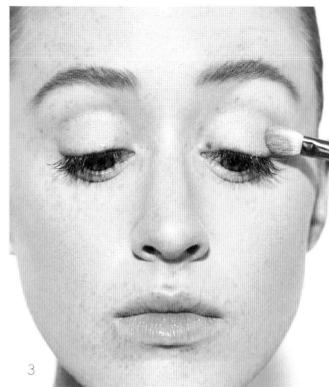

3

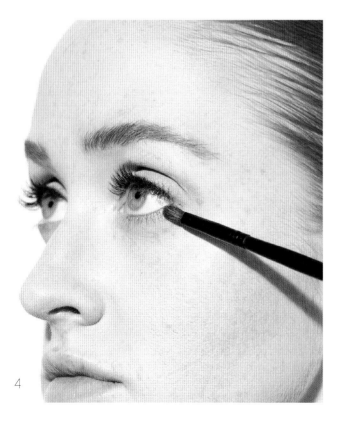

4

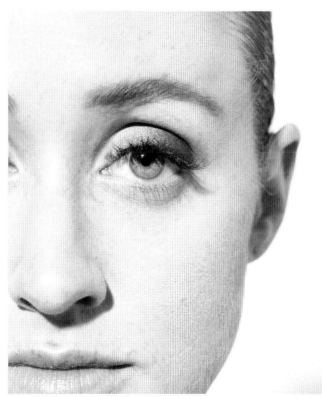

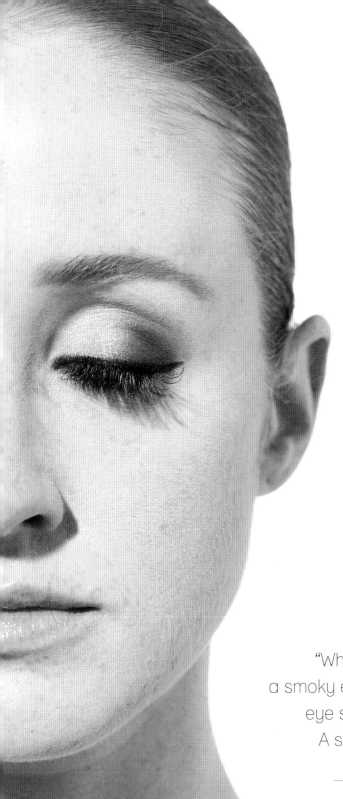

how to get a smoky eye

1. Follow *The Fiery Eye* process (page 208).

2. Apply your smoky eye shadow color of choice along the crease and lid. We love NARS Cosmetics' palette called *And God Created the Woman*. It has all of the colors you need in one easy package.

3. Blend with a soft brush.

4. Apply a nude shimmering color to your brow bone. This will accentuate the highest point on your face and bring out your features.

5. Blend more. The goal is to take away any harsh lines to give it a smoky effect.

6. Take a white shimmering shadow and apply it to the inner part of your eyelid. This will make your eyes appear wider, brighter and fresher.

7. Blend even more.

8. Using a black liquid liner, sweep a line from the inside of the eye outward.

The look is complete!

"What a lot of people misunderstand about a smoky eye is that many think it's about black or grey eye shadow engulfing the entire eye. It's not. A smokey eye is a technique not a color."

—Stephen Dimmick, redhead makeup artist

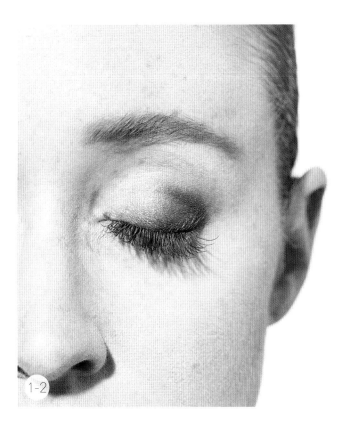

1-2

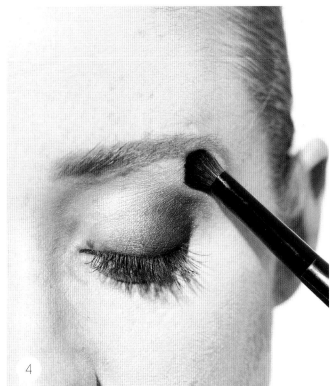

4

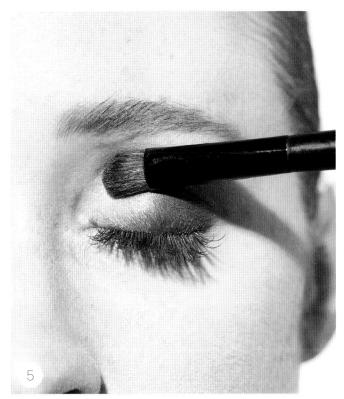

5

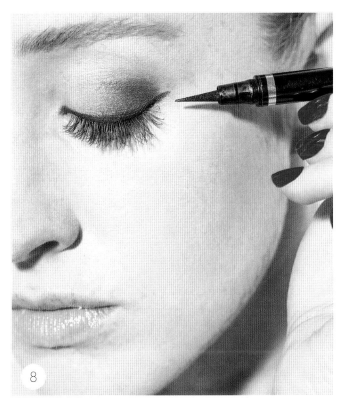

8

eyeliner

Redheads in Hollywood, like Rita Hayworth and Lucille Ball, set the bar for the most classic redhead look in history: cat-eye eyeliner and red hair. It will forever be a look every woman with red hair can turn to.

"Look at some of the most beautiful and fiercely talented women of our time: Julianne Moore, Amy Adams, Nicole Kidman, Tilda Swinton, Jessica Rabbit, to name a few. All redheads. They embraced their signature red hair. Historically, some of the most powerful and influential women are said to have been redheads. Helen of Troy, Aphrodite, Queen Elizabeth I. The moment you accept your uniqueness, it will empower you through the world."

—Christiane Seidel, actress

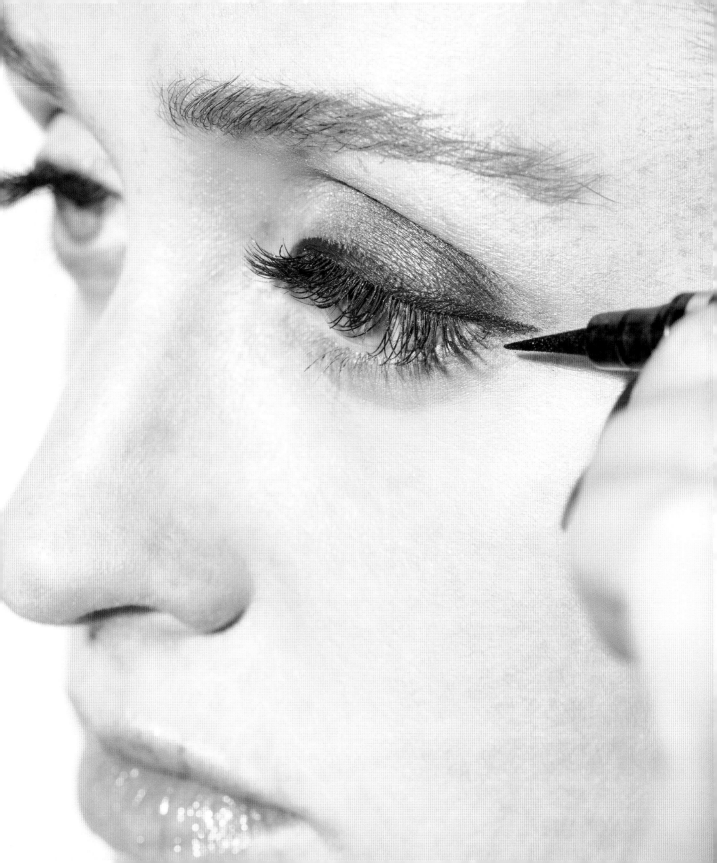

liquid, pencil or gel?

Deciding to use liquid, pencil or gel eyeliner is a personal preference. Some redheads like a pencil and gel because of the smudged look, although many redheads enjoy liquid eyeliner because it creates a more set look.

pencil

self-sharpened

Requires a pencil sharpener to create a pointed tip at the end.

our "redhead friendly" favorites

$: Revlon Photoready Kajal Eye Pencil in Matte Charcoal

$$: MAC Cosmetics Pro Longwear Eye Liner

twist up pencil

Does not require a pencil sharpener. Just twist up and apply. Make sure to purchase a twist up pencil that has a bonus blender tip at the end. The blender tip will give you the ability to smudge the liner to create a natural look.

our "redhead friendly" favorites

$: Rimmel London Exaggerate Full Colour Eye Definer

$$: Clinique Quickliner For Eyes

liquid

Liquid eyeliner is great for achieving a precise, long-lasting line. Use this type when looking to create a cat-eye.

our "redhead friendly" favorites

$: Maybelline Line Stiletto Ultimate Precision Liquid Eyeliner

$$: stila Stay All Day Waterproof Liquid Eye Liner

(3)

gel

Gel-based formula that comes in a small round pot and needs a small angled brush to apply.

our "redhead friendly" favorites

$: L'Oréal Paris Infallible Lacquer Liner 24H Eyeliner

$$: Bobbi Brown Long-Wear Gel Eyeliner

Tip #1: Have fun with eyeliner colors! Redheads look great in black, brown, green, blue and violet.

Tip #2: To make your eyes pop, use a white eyeliner on the lower waterline and inner corners of your eye.

how to apply

1. With a steady hand, apply liner as close to the lash line as possible. Start from the inside and work your way out. Or, start from the middle and work outward, lining the inside at the very end.

2. Start with a thin line in order to build up, if you wish to make it thicker.

3. If you see blonde lashes peaking through, fill in the liner directly on the root of the lashes.

4. Going for a cat-eye look? We wear a cat eye every single day. It is our signature look. Extend the liner where the lashes end. Don't pull eyelid outward. For a natural cat-eye look, draw on the liner as you are looking straight into the mirror.

5. Make a wing on the outer corner of each eye. Use your finger to dab any mistakes away and soften the line. Blend, blend, blend.

Tip #3: If you don't have a steady hand, first line eyes with a pencil, then go over it with liquid liner. This will ensure a straight and concise line.

For travelers and those on the go, applying eyeliner with eye shadow is a great recommendation.

how to apply

1. Apply eye shadow primer.

2. Damp an angled brush with a bit of water and dip it into the eyeliner color of choice. It is best to go with black or brown. But if you're daring, you can opt for greens and blues.

3. Hold skin tight by gently placing the index finger where the lashes end and pulling outward.

4. Apply the eyeliner starting from the inside corner and going all the way to the end. This will ensure you achieve a straight, easy-to-blend line.

5. Use a cotton swab to clean any areas where the eye shadow may have fallen, mainly under the eye.

Tip #4: We highly suggest not lining the entire eye or the rim of the eyelid. It can make the eyes appear very small.

"False eyelashes can be tricky, but look incredible on redheads because redheads tend to have light-colored fine lashes. False eyelashes add length and density to the lash line, which in effect makes the eyes look bigger, doe-eyed and awake. Individual lashes look the most natural but require a little more patience and dexterity."

—Lauren Gott, redhead makeup artist

fake eyelashes

Everyone has something that gives them an extra boost of confidence, maybe your fabulous red hair, a certain outfit, super high heels or a manicure, but fake lashes are it for both of us. We've been playing around with lashes for many years now, and here's a few thoughts and tips to consider if you are thinking about getting into the lashes game.

full vs. individual lashes

full lashes

1. Full Strip Natural Lashes

These false lashes are more natural looking and give a slight boost in length and thickness. These are great for daytime outings.

2. Full Strip Thick Lashes

These lashes are much thicker looking than the natural lashes. While these lashes may look too heavy for everyday wear, they are actually great for photos.

3. Full Strip Long and Short Lashes

This category of lashes has a bold pattern of longer and shorter lashes. This is a more dramatic look.

individual lashes

These are the favorite among false eyelash lovers. Instead of getting lashes together in a strip, these come in different lengths and are attached individually until the lash line is full. These lashes do take longer to put on, but they look more natural where your eyelid meets your lash line (you avoid the strip that holds traditional false lashes together) and you can put on as many or as few as you want to customize your length and look.

how to apply individual eyelashes

1. Apply eyelash glue to the back of the hand and allow it to dry and become slightly tacky, about 10 seconds.

2. Use a pair of tweezers to grasp the individual false lash by the lash flair, leaving the base free.

3. Dip the eyelash base in the glue and start by laying the base on the natural lash line from the outside of the eye and working inward, side by side. Sometimes we just add lashes to the outside edges of the eye to create a winged effect.

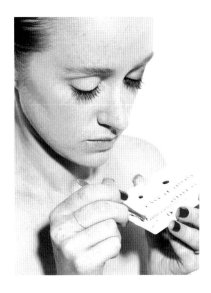
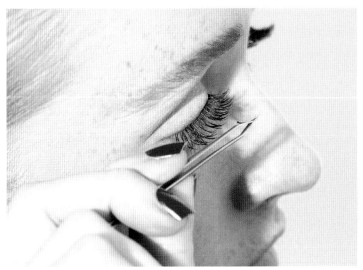

how to apply full-set eyelashes

A full set can be used by measuring the false lashes with the natural eyelash line and trimming according to the size of the eye.

1. The false set doesn't need to go all the way to the inside edge of the eye. The inside edge of a false set will often lift away if it's too close.

2. Apply eyelash glue to the back of the hand and allow it to dry and become slightly tacky.

3. Use a pointed cotton swab to apply the glue from the hand to the base of the false lashes.

4. Start laying the full lash set from the outside edge of the eye inward.

5. Grasp the full set and your natural lashes and squeeze them together slightly.

6. Open the eye and apply a little pressure by tapping lashes at the base to ensure they are secure and laying nicely.

Good glue makes a *world* of a difference. You will not be a very happy redhead if your lashes keep falling off, right? Follow the instructions on the back of the box and remember to always let the glue set on the false lashes for about 30 seconds before attaching the lash to your lid—this little tip will help a lot because the glue is more sticky (and easier to adhere) as it begins to dry. Make sure to *always* keep a spare tube of adhesive, tweezers and some spare lashes in your makeup bag when you wear falsies. You definitely don't want to be stuck without a fix-it kit if something doesn't stick right the first time.

our "redhead friendly" favorites

$: Duo Eyelash Adhesive in Clear

$: Ardell Brush-On Latex-free Lash Adhesive *(great for super sensitive eyes)*

step 6. confidence—
empowering eyebrows

"Don't ask a redhead with perfectly shaped eyebrows why she is late."

Natural redheads usually have fair eyebrows, but there are the select few who have naturally darker brows. Either way, it's very important to shape and fill in the brow to give the eyes and face definition. It's also essential to care for the eyebrow hair because a redhead's brows are typically coarse. Learning how to brush the brow upward and using the right products can transform the face from *BLEAK to FLEEK!*

"Eyebrows are sisters, not twins."

There are so many different types of eyebrow products, but here are our "redhead friendly" favorites.

pencil: self-sharpened

$$: Clinique SuperFine Liner For Brows

$$: Regular Pencil: Benefit Cosmetics Instant Brow Pencil

powder

$: Nyx Cosmetics Eyebrow Cake Powder in Auburn/Red

$$: Youngblood Brow Artiste in Auburn

"Nature knows what it's doing. If a gal's brows are fine and dainty, keep with that shape. Fuller brows should stay around that. The brows are the frames to the eye. They should add framing, but not overpower. You want a brow shade that will enhance, but not overpower your brow hairs. Don't get too caught up in matching your hair. Generally, it looks most natural for brows to be a tone lighter than the hair. This makes the eyes the darkest feature on the face and softens it."

—Brett Freedman, makeup artist and owner/creator
of Brett Freedman Beauty

"Be careful what you do to your eyebrows. And please don't go MAROON in hopes of enhancing what God gave ya. Nobody looks good in maroon. Including (especially?) the members of Maroon 5."

—Julie Klausner, Duchess of Comedy

gel

Eyebrow gel lifts and holds while keeping the brow hairs in place. There are two types of appropriate eyebrow gels: clear and tinted. Redheads can really benefit from using a tinted eyebrow gel, because it grooms the brow while giving them a hint of natural color. It's best to find one that has a rich auburn shade and adds fullness to brows.

Tinted gel is also an option for those who do not want to dye their eyebrow hair, because it will give them the same (yet temporary) effect.

how to apply

Apply eyebrow gel in upward strokes in the direction of your hair growth. You can apply the gel product alone or together with a pencil or eyebrow powder.

our "redhead friendly" favorites

Clear Eyebrow Gel: Urban Decay Brow Tamer Flexible Hold Brow Gel

Tinted Eyebrow Gel: Tarte Colored Clay Tinted Brow Gel in Taupe

Tip #1: If you prefer a more set look, find a product that has an angled bristled brush to get into the hard-to-reach areas of the brow, like the arch and ends.

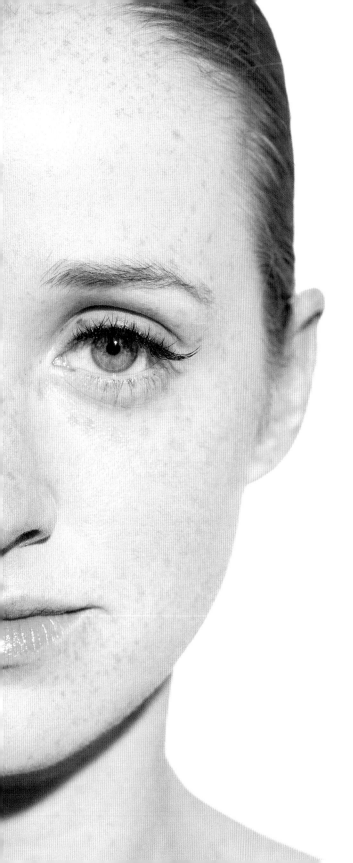

how to fill in
eyebrows properly

This should be the last step in a makeup routine because foundation and powder residue can land on the brows. You want to ensure the eyebrows look clean and polished.

1. Using a spoolie brush, comb and brush brows in upward strokes. Trim and tweeze brows if needed.

2. Apply the eyebrow product of choice (pencil and/ or powder) lightly, concentrating on the arch because it lifts the eye. Make sure to fill in any sparse areas to make the eyebrow look full.

3. Next, use a spoolie brush to gently blend and remove any excess product.

4. Lastly, using a tinted eyebrow gel or clear eyebrow gel, brush the eyebrow upward once more. The gel will lock in the look.

Optional: You have the option of skipping steps 2 to 4 and simply use a tinted eyebrow gel as recommended on page 225. It was designed to fill in the brows with a natural tint, give definition and lock in the color instantly. The above steps are for a more glamorized *wow* look.

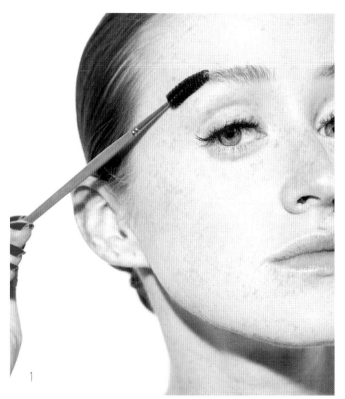

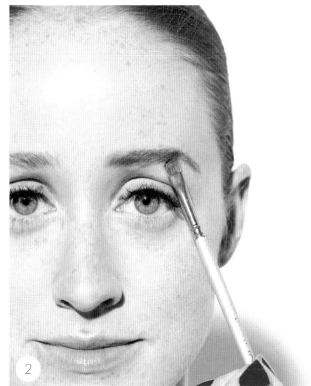

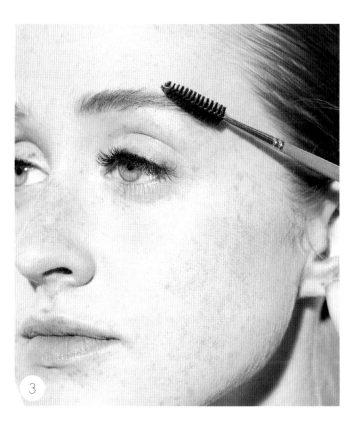

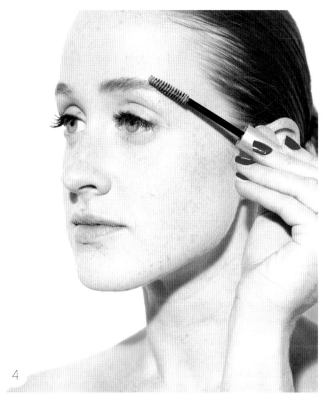

how to trim eyebrows

"I like to brush brow hairs up and trim just the tips. Then brush hairs down and do the same. Brush back and assess. If it still feels like they are long, brush up and down again and snip a little more off. Always do this in tiny trims, so you can avoid over trimming and have the dreaded 'nubs' that stick straight out. You do want the brows to have a natural lilt."

—Brett Freedman, makeup artist and owner/creator
of Brett Freedman Beauty

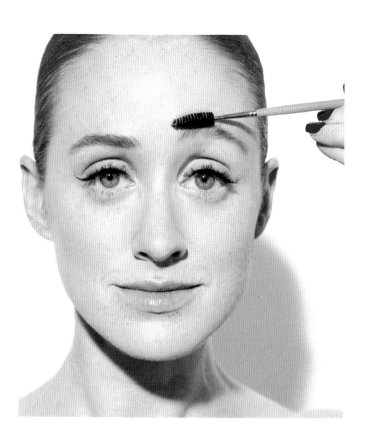
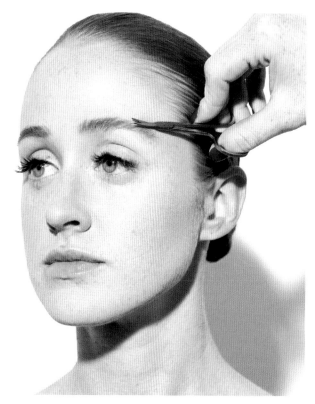

So how do you know where your brows should begin and end?

Place a tweezer or straight object (like a pencil) vertically on the outer edge of the brow, alongside the nose. The point where it lands at the brow marks the beginning of your eyebrow. Then, place the object parallel to the outside corner of your iris; this is where your arch should be. Then angle it from your nostril to the outside of the brow; that is where the eyebrow should end.

how to tweeze properly

We love thick eyebrows. Period. Thicker shaped eyebrows frame the face better and are much easier to maintain and fill in. Be sure to never overtweeze the eyebrow hair. Only tweeze the stray hairs outside the brow's natural shape or have a professional esthetician shape the eyebrows to best suit your face shape. Keeping in line with the tips above, gently tweeze hair a row or two from the brow for a natural look. It's always better to tweeze less than more. Do not overpluck!

You also have the option of using an eyebrow stencil to help instantly find the start, arch and ending point of your eyebrows. Then, simply fill in the eyebrow using the stencil as a guide.

our "redhead friendly" favorite

$$: Anastasia Beverly Hills Stencils

Using an eyebrow highlighter on the brow bone enhances the arch and adds definition to brows.

1. After filling in brows, trace a line underneath the brow from the beginning to the end.

2. Blend with finger.

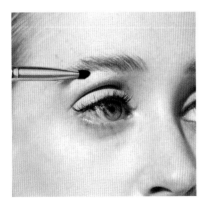 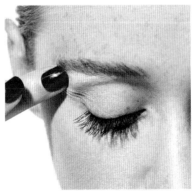 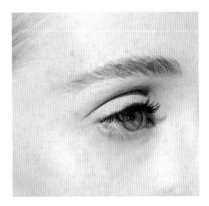

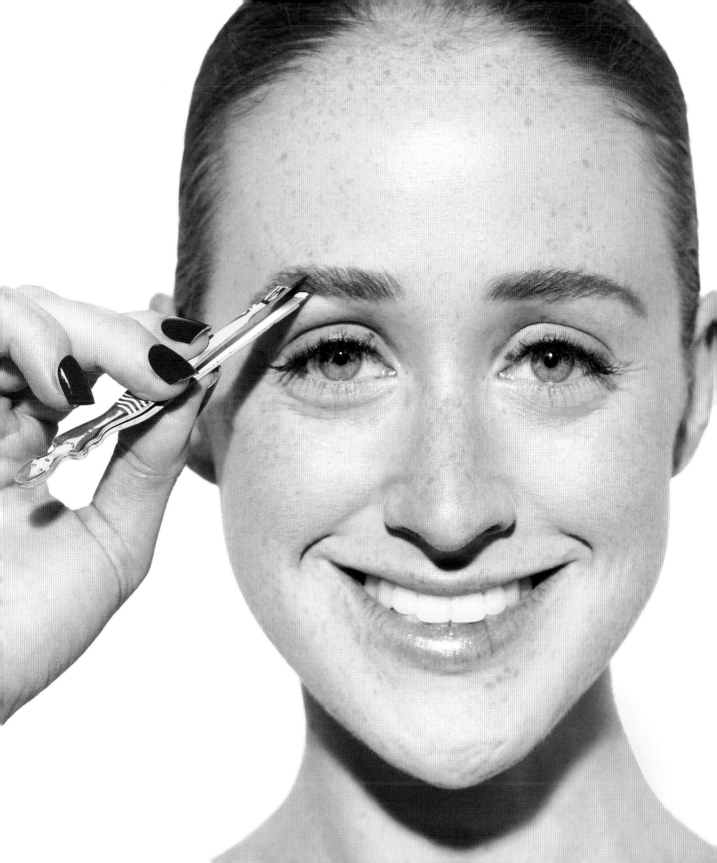

eyebrow and eyelash tinting

Instead of investing a lot of time applying and reapplying eyebrow product, many women adore eyelash and eyebrow tinting, especially those with fair brows. Honestly who wants to put on mascara and pencil if you don't have to? Although eyelash and eyebrow tinting has hit the mainstream, many redheads haven't tried them. Here are a few tips to see if eyelash tinting is right for you.

Eyelash Tinting: We always recommend visiting an esthetician. Eyes are very sensitive and need extra care, and a professional will be able to give you the best natural-looking color for your skin tone and hair shade. It's about $20 to $30 each and lasts for three to six weeks. Redheads can choose to do black or brown.

Eyebrow Tinting: For light eyebrows, use a tint that is a shade or two darker. This will complement the skin and leave eyebrows looking natural and full.

permanent eyebrows (also known as eyebrow tattooing)

Instead of shopping around for eyebrow products or getting the brows temporarily dyed, many opt for eyebrow tattooing. Unfortunately, some women have ended up with terrible results. That's why the number one tip is to find an eyebrow expert who has many years of experience with tattooing eyebrows. Ask to look at their past work to ensure results are natural looking. Invest money in selecting the right technician and choose an eyebrow color based on skin tone and hair shade.

from day to party

At this point, steps 1 through 6 should be your daytime look. You can quickly transform your look to night by following steps 7 and 8.

step 7. bronzer and blush— it's okay to use them!

The next step is bronzer and blush. Society has told redheads not to use blush or bronzer, but society, you are wrong! Redheads look great in bronzers and blushes, no matter if you have freckles, fair or dark skin.

"I prefer to use both a blush and bronzer. The bronzer should be used first. It will give you your contour but make sure it is matte!"

—Flynn Marie Pyykkonen, makeup artist

bronzer

The purpose of this product is to give the skin some color while highlighting the cheekbones and giving the effect of a natural, safe tan. Don't make the mistake (like Adrienne did as a teenager) of dramatically piling on dark bronzer. The idea is to make it look natural and subtly sun kissed.

Powder Bronzer: comes in a compact case.

our "redhead friendly" favorite

$$: tarte Amazonian Clay

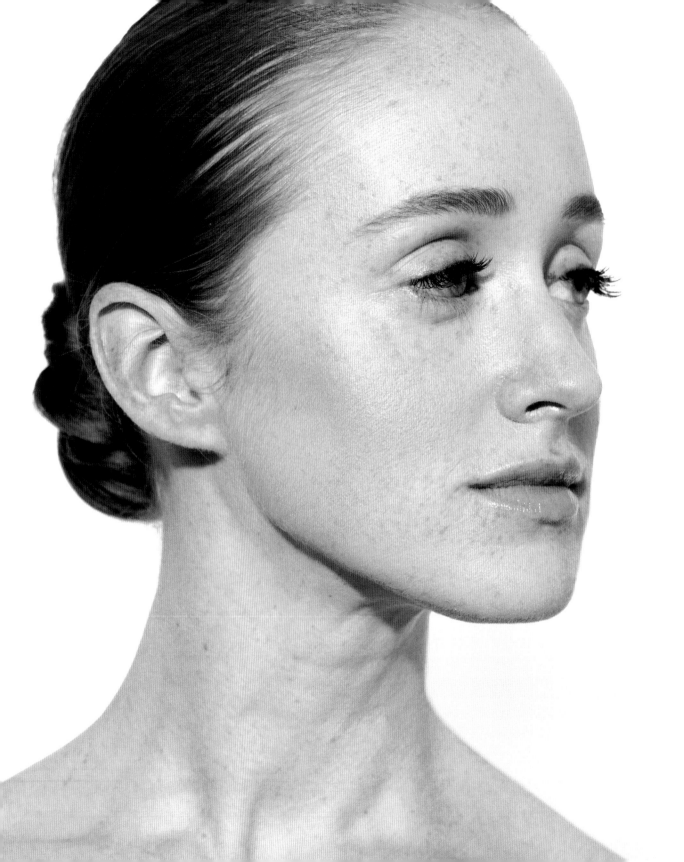

Mineral Bronzer: comes in the form of powder.

our "redhead friendly" favorite

$$: Lancôme "Star Bronzer" Magic Bronzing Brush

how to apply

Using a bronzer brush, create the number "3" on both sides of your face. Start at the top of the forehead, dust it along your cheeks and sweep it around the jawline all the way to your chin. Remember to blend into the neck. Keep in mind that a bronzer should only be one to two shades darker than skin tone.

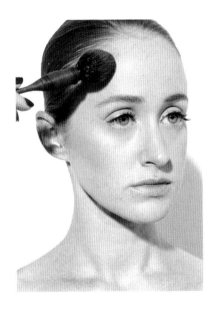
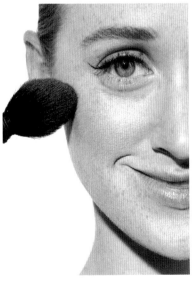
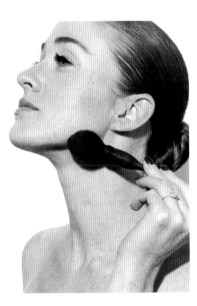

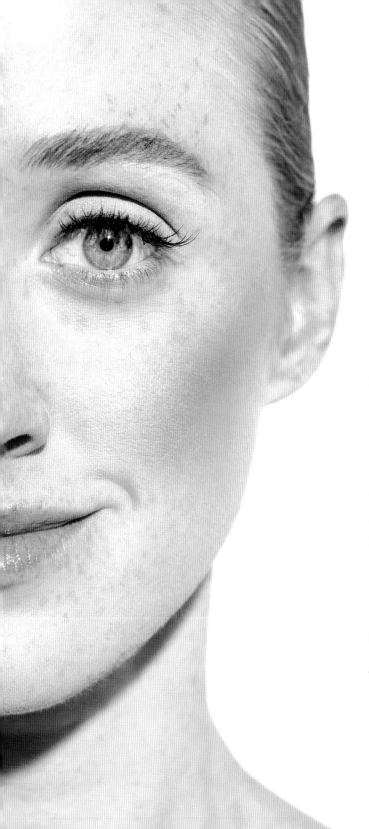

blush

Known as *rouge* in France and blusher in the UK, blush is used to give a natural "blushing effect" to the cheeks and to emphasize cheekbones. It has been widely taught that redheads cannot wear blush because the pink tones will clash with red hair. But this could not be more wrong. Like most "redhead friendly" products, it is all about finding the right color blush for you. Usually, deeper blushes are best for redheads with fair skin and freckles.

how to apply

1. Lightly sweep a medium-size blush brush on the product and tap it to remove any excess. If you're using a cream or gel, dab a little on the ring finger.

2. Do a fish face, and apply the blush. This will help you find the apple of the cheeks because the apples are the round rises where you naturally blush.

3. Apply the blush to the center of the apples. If using a cream or gel, dot the color first, then use your finger or a makeup sponge to blend in.

4. Remember: Less is always more!

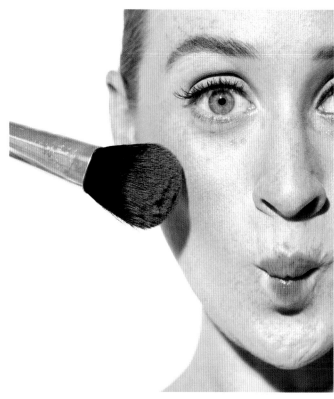

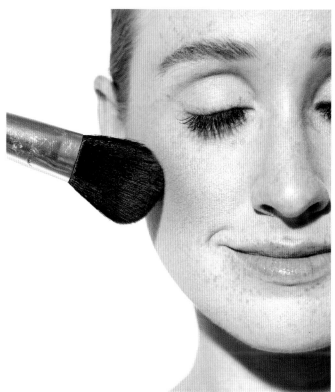

our "redhead friendly" favorites

powder

$$: MAC Cosmetics Powder Blush
in Gingerly

cream

$$: Cargo Swimmables Water Resistant
Blush in Los Cabos

mineral

$$: Youngblood Mineral Cosmetics Crushed
Mineral Blush

Always use a makeup brush!
Avoid using cotton balls or powder
puffs as these do not work well
to blend in color.

highlighters and illuminators

These add a little pop of shine to makeup.

Highlighters: Gives a glow-y, shimmery look. Apply to cheekbones, avoiding the T-zone at all times.

our "redhead friendly" favorite

$$$: BECCA Beach Tint Shimmer Soufflé

Illuminators: Gives a dewy look. Apply to cheekbones over/under makeup or mix product with liquid foundation.

our "redhead friendly" favorite

$$: Benefit Cosmetics High Beam Face Highlighter

step 8. glamorous lips

Many redheads think they cannot wear a bright lip because their hair is vibrant. When we were younger, we would wear nude shades to blend in with the crowd, and we soon found we were missing out. Redheads looks absolutely stunning with a bright, bold lip. No matter the season or shade of red hair, a bold lip makes hair pop even more.

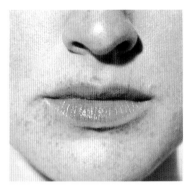
Lip Gloss

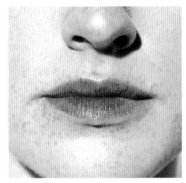
Lip Stain

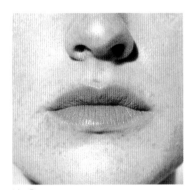
Lip Crayon

different types of lip products for your everyday red life

Lip gloss: Gives lips a glossy finish.

Lip stain: Gives lips a matte, natural finish.

Lipstick: Gives lips a solid color finish.

Lip crayon: Lipstick in the form of a crayon.

Lip liner: Product used to outline lips.

Lip balm: Product used to moisturize lips.

Lip oil: An oil-based lip balm that moisturizes and smoothens lips.

choosing the right lip color

Redheads can wear every color, trust us! Oranges, plums, reds and pinks—we love them all.

Here is a guide to our all-time favorite lip shades and brands.

"NARS Lipstick in 'Mindgame' is the perfect complement to my auburn hair. A sheer brandy, it gives my look a monochrome feel."

—Jessica Matlin, deputy beauty editor at *Cosmopolitan* magazine

hair shade	strawberry blonde	copper	classic red	deep red
light complexion (fair/ porcelain)	$$$: Mary Kay Creme Lipstick in "Sweet Nectar"	$$$: Tory Burch Lip Color in "Pretty Baby"	$$$: Ellis Faas Glazed Lips L301 in "Ellis Red"	$$$: Dior Rouge Dior #999 in "Ara Red"* *great for all redheads
medium/dark complexion (olive skin)	$: Revlon Super Lustrous Lipstick in "Gentlemen Prefer Pink"	$$: MAC Cosmetics Sheen Supreme Lipstick in "Good to be Bad"	$: Sephora Collection Rouge Shine Lipstick in No. 19 "V.I.P Shimmer"	$: CoverGirl Continuous Color Lipstick 770 in "Bronze Glow"

hair shade	auburn	deep auburn	red violet
light complexion (fair/ porcelain)	$$: Make Up For Ever Rouge Artist Intense Color Lipstick in 40 "Satin Bright Orange"	$$$: Chanel Rouge Allure in 98 "Coromandel"	$$: Hourglass Cosmetics Femme Rouge Velvet Crème in "Fresco"
medium/dark complexion (olive skin)	$: Revlon Super Lustrous Lipstick in "Gentlemen Prefer Pink"	$$$: Yves Saint Laurent Glossy Stain Rebel Nudes in "Nude Provocateur"	$$: stila Color Balm Lipstick in "Isla"

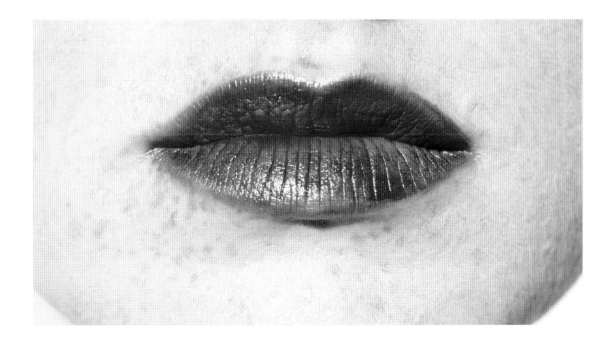

light complexion (fair/porcelain) redheads

This type of redhead tends to have a cool tone and should stick to lip colors with blue or purple undertones. Lean toward bold colors such as pink, red, mauve and orange. This way your pale complexion will shine, giving you a pop of color.

medium/dark complexion (olive skin) redheads

This type of redhead tends to have be warm toned and should stick to lip colors with a yellow undertone. Lean toward bright and rich shades such as orange red, coral, tangerine, cranberry and deep plum.

"redhead friendly" lip color tips

1. Brighter hue hair colors should look for blue undertone lip colors.

2. Golden reds and auburn hair colors should look for yellow undertone and warm lip colors.

3. Don't match the shade of lipstick to your hair color or you'll look super washed out.

4. The best tip for redheads is to go with a warmer shade of a particular color. So with pink, go for a deep pink, like a pink orchid.

5. Don't be afraid of nude! When your eyes are bold and strong, a nude lip pulls the look together perfectly. But do not rock this shade if your eyes are bare; the contrast will not complement your hair.

how to achieve the perfect red lip

In order to prevent smudging, applying a "redhead friendly" lipstick should be the last step in the makeup routine. Think of it as the final touch to a painting. A fun lip color is easy to achieve, but here are the steps to achieve a perfect red lip:

1. Start with completely bare lips. Apply a lip base (we always recommend a lip balm) to avoid dryness. If your lips are extra dry, apply a lip scrub first (page 120).

2. Use a lip liner that complements the chosen lip shade. Lip liners will prolong lip color and make lips look fuller. Choose a lip liner that is the same color, or a little lighter, than the lipstick color.

Tip #1: There is no need to splurge on a liner. The standard lip liners
from a local drugstore will do the trick.

3. Line the entire perimeter of the lip. Don't worry if you mess up and get an uneven line because the lipstick will fix it. Using a tissue, gently rub the mistake off the skin and add a dab of foundation to the spot. Rub the foundation into the skin to cover any imperfections.

Tip #2: Try not to fill in the lip solely with lip liner. Redheads suffer
from sensitive skin, and the liner will dry out the lips if a moisturizer
or lipstick isn't applied afterward.

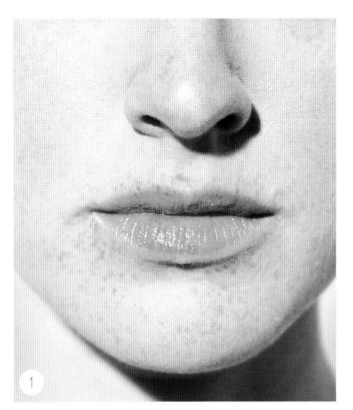

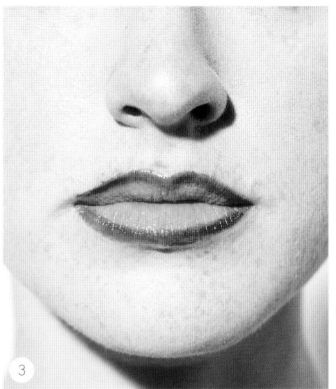

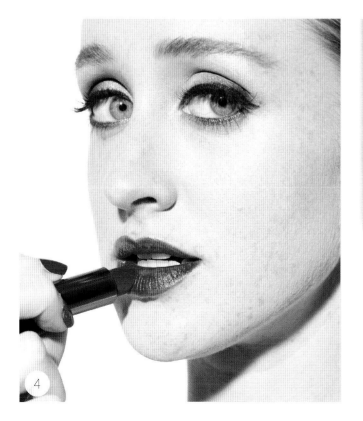

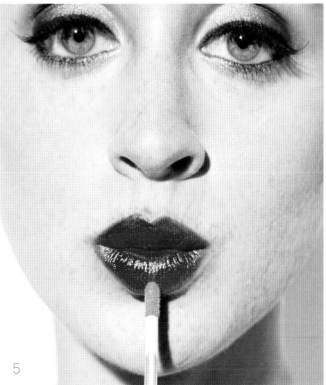

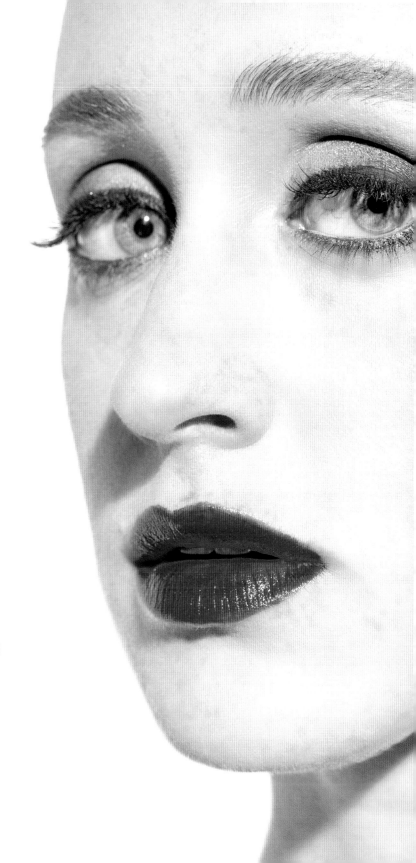

4. Grab your lipstick and glide it over the lips. Trace the entire lip. If you happen to miss and get lipstick on the skin, don't rub it or else it will blend into the skin and create a reddish look. Simply dip a cotton swab into makeup remover and wipe off the lipstick.

5. Now that lips are done, apply a gloss. This enhances the color even more. The type of gloss can be clear, pink or red. We recommend choosing a gloss color similar to the chosen lipstick color.

6. To set the lipstick, place a tissue over the lips and press down. To make sure it does not get on the teeth, make an "O" shape with the lips. While mouth is open, put your (clean!) index finger directly in the mouth and pull out. You'll see excess on the finger. This is the stuff that would normally land on the front teeth.

7. Take lip liner, lipstick and gloss with you wherever you go (depending on how lasting the lipstick is) because you will need to reapply. If your lipstick is long lasting, simply take your lip liner and gloss.

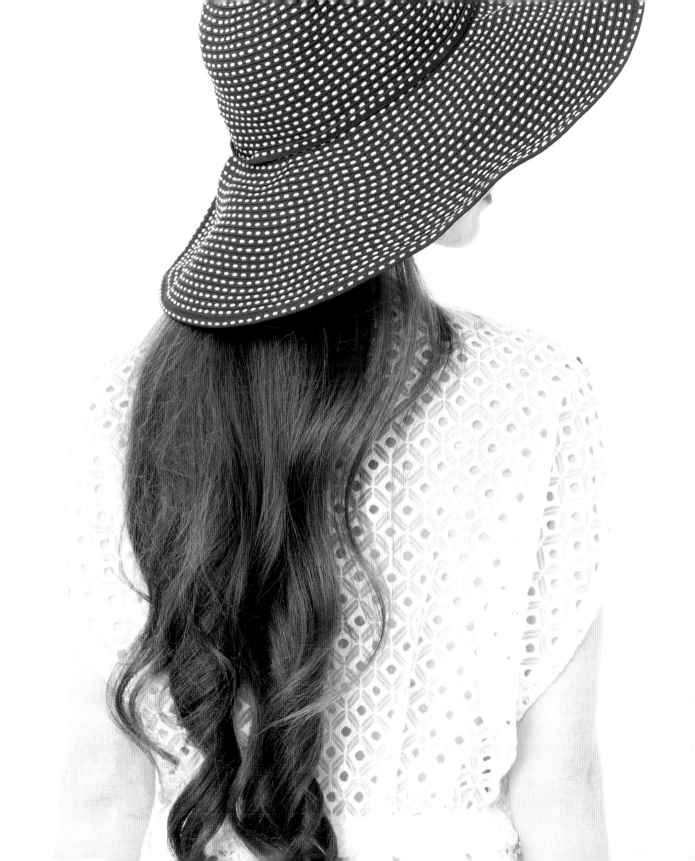

get the celebrity look

"Jessica Chastain and Julianne Moore opened the door for redheads. When they became famous in Hollywood, redheads started to get more attention. It used to be so rare to find editorial models with red hair. In the last few years, you've seen more and more. But redhead celebrities have made everyone all say, 'Wow! Redheads ARE beautiful.'"

—Felicia Milewicz, ex-beauty director of *Glamour* magazine for 40 years

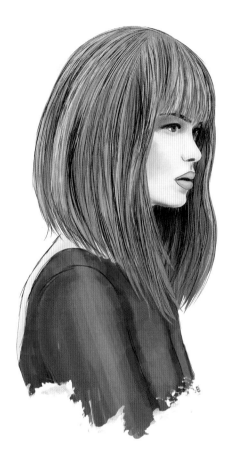

a daring hairstyle for every redhead, by Nick Arrojo, owner and founder of ARROJO NYC

"My favorite haircut of all time is a graduated bob cut with a razor and I think it's perfect for sassy redheads. Visually, there are a variety of reasons to love a graduated razor-cut bob. The graduation from the occipital bone to the nape helps to *elevate* the hair, giving body and fullness and flirty-ness."

how to style the look

1. A smooth blow-dry and some flatiron action will create a sleek, shiny, elongated version.

2. A round brush, curling iron or wand lets you create lots of full and sexy tousles, with tumbling swing and movement.

This cut is especially beneficial for redheads with thick and/or coarse hair because of the weight removal.

Reba-inspired red carpet makeup glam, by Brett Freedman, Reba McEntire's makeup artist

1. Foundation: Start with a sheer tinted moisturizer, like Laura Mercier Tinted Moisturizer in Nude. Apply to entire face, under jaw and neck. "Reba's freckles are light, so they rarely show through even the sheerest foundation. I wish they did. I love them!"

2. Under Eye: Use a touch of concealer on lids and in inner eyes to even out and brighten. Brett uses Clé de Peau Beauté Concealer in Light.

3. Face Powder: Set the makeup with a loose powder, like Make Up For Ever's Super Matte Loose Powder in Sand. The super matte powder helps balance the moisturizing face tint.

4. Cheeks: Use apricot and peachy shades on the cheeks. Brett loves MAC Cosmetics Powder Blushes in peachy tones. Next, glisten the cheeks with a highlighter, like It Cosmetics Hello Light Powder Illuminizer. This will give the skin depth.

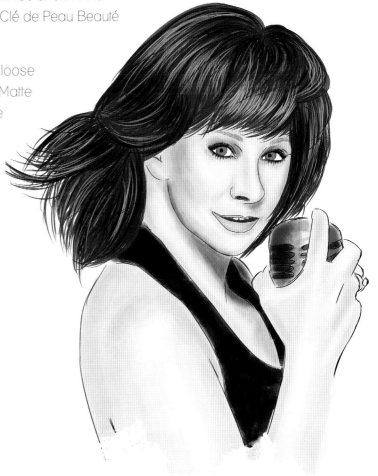

5. Eye Shadow: Mix warm and cool tones to make your eyes pop. Brett uses Urban Decay's nude palettes in the crease, bottom lash line and brow bone. Next, using a damp brush, he applies MAC Cosmetics Eye Shadow in Idol Eyes shadow to the top lid and inner eye. This technique turns a shimmer shadow into a creme shadow.

6. Eyeliner: Apply a dark liner on top of the lash line. This will give life to the eye and add drama. Brett uses tarte's Tarteist Clay Paint Liner in black. Next, use a deep shadow crisply on the bottom lash line.

7. Lashes: Curl lashes with a lash curler, like Shu Uemura's Eyelash Curler. Then apply mascara. Apply three coats to the upper lashes and two to the bottom. Brett loves L'Oréal Voluminous Carbon Black Volume Building Mascara. Once dry, press very softly to pop up lashes and align.

8. Brow: Brett always struggled to find the right products for Reba's ginger toned eyebrows. So, he created his own line called Brett Brow. His Mono Shade brow pencils come in two redhead shades, Auburnista and Gingerella, inspired by Reba.

9. Lips: Use a neutral lip pencil to fill in the entire lip, like Rimmel London Lasting Finish 1000 Kisses Lip Liner. Next, wake up the lips with a bold lipstick or gloss.

Julianne Moore's red carpet twisted updo, by Marcus Francis, Julianne's hairstylist

You'll need: Thickening spray, mousse, blow dryer, bobby pins

1. On damp hair, apply a thickening spray at the roots and comb through.

2. Use a large dollop of mousse to cover the hair from roots to ends and comb through.

3. Determine which side you want to part and blow-dry the hair straight with a round brush.

4. Make a heavy swoop across the front as your pull the hair down and back.

5. With one hand, begin twisting, starting at the nape of the neck. Using hairpins, begin to secure the twist to the head. Continue twisting the rest of the hair, going toward the crown and pinning along the way to secure your progress.

6. Tuck the ends inside the twist using bobby pins to secure. Make sure to leave some height at the crown.

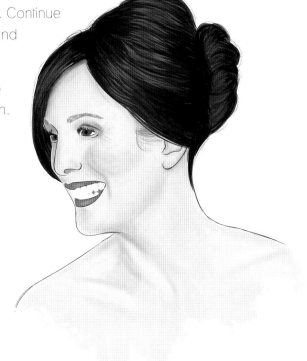

"My biggest red carpet accomplishment was doing Julianne Moore's side-swept chignon for her Best Actress win at the Oscars. Julianne Moore usually prefers classic, as well as relaxed, hair for red-carpet events. Her hair texture is pretty similar to that of most redheads: thick, healthy and strong."

Joan from *Mad Men*'s 6Os bouffant hairstyle, by Terrie v. Owen, Christina Hendricks's hairstylist on AMC's *Mad Men*

Terrie is the master behind Christina Hendricks's bouffant look in the TV series *Mad Men*.

You'll need: Teasing comb, boar bristle brush, setting spray, texture styling creme and hot rollers.

1. This look is for medium length or longer. If you don't have much hair, don't be afraid to pop in hairpieces to add bulk and length. Visit your local wig salons and they will give you options for modern, cute hairpieces and extensions.

2. Always set the hair going back and away from the face. Tease the hair at the root BEFORE you put the rollers in. This gives you massive volume and holds for hours. Never take a section of hair that's bigger than the roller. Spray setting lotion only at the root, just one pump, and do not spray the whole section. Wrap hair in roller.

3. Use good-quality bobby pins, not the shiny ones, as they will slip out of the hair. Brush the hair out with a good boar bristle brush, gather it up into a ponytail just above the nape and give it a good twist. Then, start pinning from the nape all the way up the back until you get the desired shape. Pin up any loose ends or leave hanging for more of a modern Bridget Bardot look.

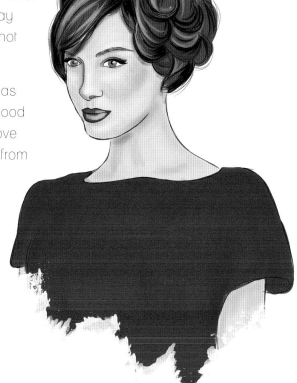

favorite beauty tips from our followers

For one month, we hosted #TipThursday on our Facebook and Instagram pages. Our "redhead beauties" shared their favorite redhead beauty tips. These were some of our favorites.

Sam via Instagram: I use baby sunscreen if I plan on being outside for a while. The sunscreen is thicker but it also works well for my pale and sensitive skin.

Rhomany via Facebook: A little smudge of purple eyeliner will set off both green eyes and freckles.

Rae M. via Instagram: Embrace your peaches and cream complexion. Don't tan if you have fair skin.

Amanda S. via Instagram: Drink tons of cucumber juice!

Heather O. via Instagram: Step outside the box when it comes to color!

Liz M. via Facebook: I put a drop of frankincense in my daily moisture. My skin has never looked so good! It has healing qualities like no other. No more dry patches, no more breakouts.... And it's even brightened and evened out my tone.

Aubri via Instagram: Clear mascara for frizzy flyalways—just twist into shape.

Erin via Instagram: My best redhead beauty tip is to make sure all your features shine! Don't overdo it on foundation or bronzer. Let the world see you in all your pale, freckly glory!

Penelope via Instagram: Keeping your inner redhead beautiful is what counts! Outer beauty is something we all have in our own way and the only way to really channel that inner beauty is by accepting that we are who we are and there is a reason for it.

#howtobearedhead

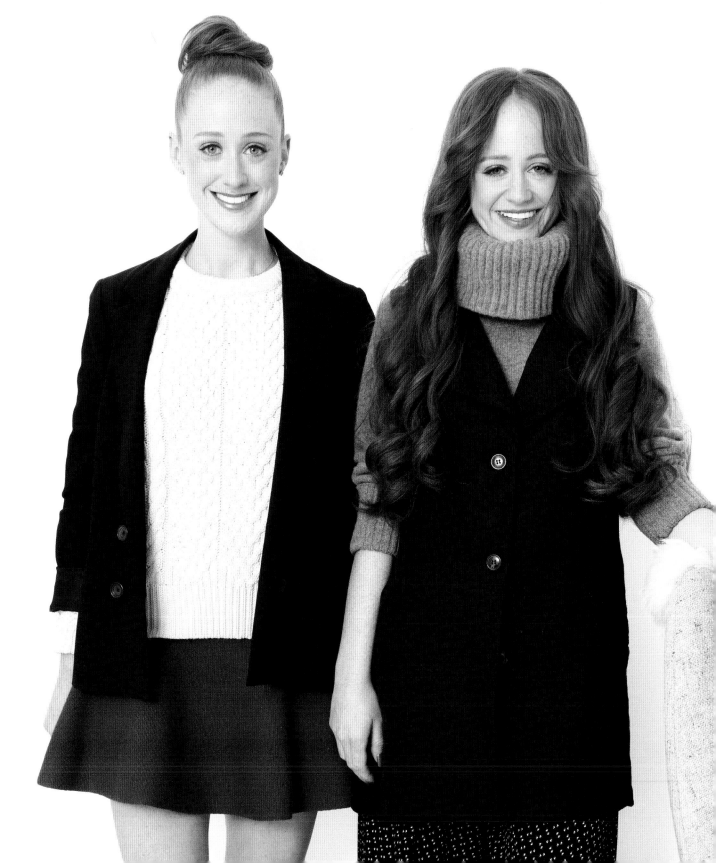

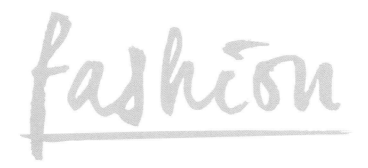

fashion

"My favorite 'redhead friendly' colors are
purple, magenta, green and blue
with a lot of violet in it."

—Nicole Miller, American fashion designer

"Wear colors like black, white, green
and purple to offset red hair."

—Margaret Nagle, screenwriter and producer

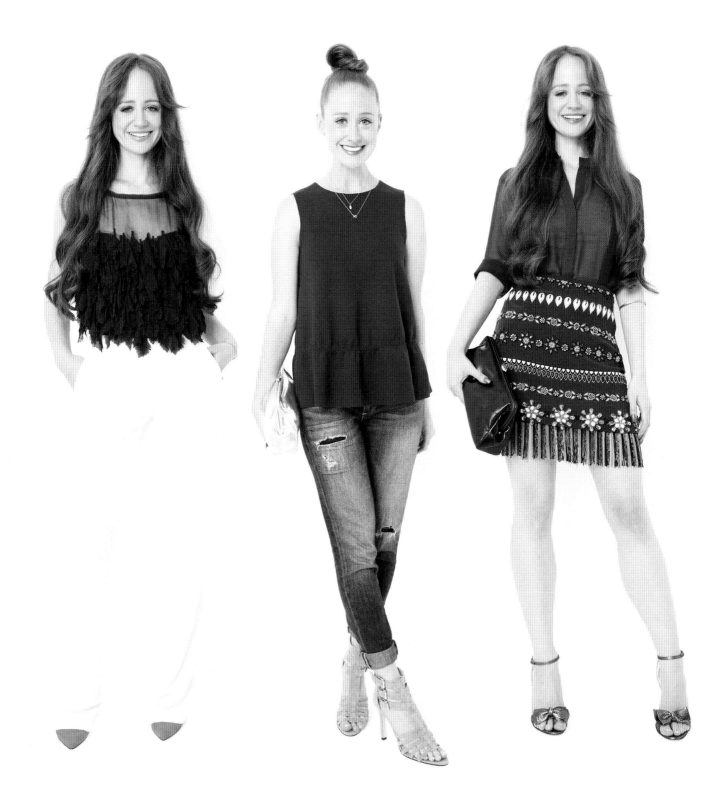

There are many myths that redheads can't wear certain colors, like pink, red, white or pastels. We solidly believe red hair complements every color, but it depends on the following: 1) The tone of a redhead's skin, 2) the shade of a redhead's hair and 3) the undertones of the fashion piece.

Our favorite colors on a redhead are those we call "redhead friendly." They are colors that enhance the features of someone with red hair.

our "redhead friendly" favorite colors

Emerald tones

Eggplant and plum purple

Sapphire, peacock and navy blue

Emerald and cast iron green

Deep cranberry

Ruby red

Mustard seed

If a redhead chooses a deeper color on the spectrum wheel, it is always a classic choice. Instead of bright red, choose a deep cranberry or ruby red. Instead of bright bird yellow, choose a mustard seed. The deeper colors are sure to give the skin and red hair a beautiful contrast. Of course, it depends on your personal look.

Here are the recommended color choices for redheads based on hair and skin tone:

	strawberry	copper	classic red	deep red	auburn	deep auburn	red violet
cool toned	Cobalt blue Aqua green/blue	Gray teal Black	Violet purple Emerald green	Radiant orchid Cranberry red	Turquoise Blue iris	Ivory Red/orange	Marsala Army green
warm toned	Pale pink Gold	Coral True red	Peach Eggshell	Light red Daffodil yellow	Champagne Pink mist	Gray lilac Candid blue	Warm red True white

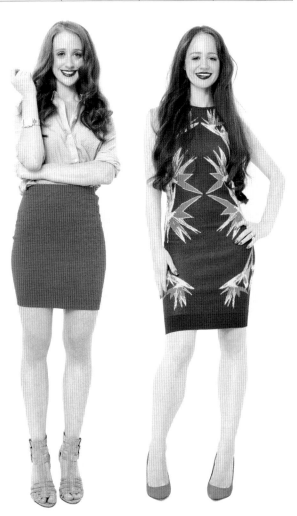

our "redhead friendly" favorite colors

spring/summer

Opt for brighter colors like fuchsia, coral and teal

Opt for warmer colors like pumpkin orange, cranberry, black, cobalt blue and emerald green

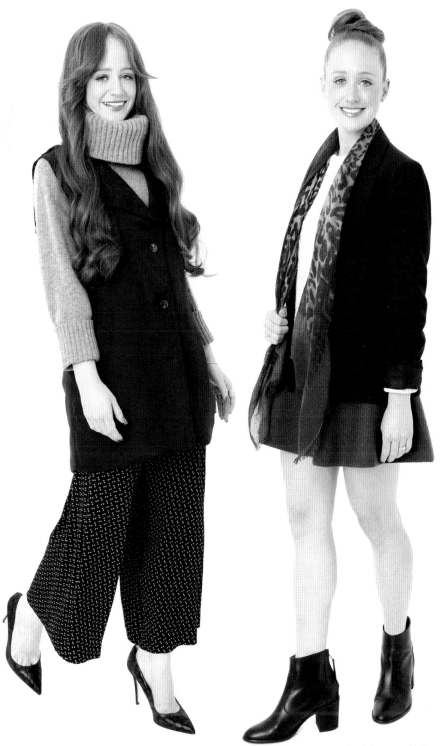

redhead myths

Many redheads think they can't wear certain colors with their red hair. Well, we're here to crack some myths that have surfaced over the last several years and explain why they're busted.

1. *Myth:* Redheads cannot wear red.

Busted: Redheads look great in red. The trick is to pick the right color red. Scarlet red is one of our favorite colors for every redhead, no matter skin tone or hair shade.

2. *Myth:* Redheads can't wear white.

Busted: It is true that fair skin paired with white may cause the skin to look washed out. But we encourage white on white. The best tip is to wear creamy white over a bright white. For instance, pair a white tank top with an ivory/off-white jean jacket. When wearing white, always make sure to make the makeup a bit more intense—deeper eyes and a touch of bronzer on the cheeks.

3. *Myth:* Redheads can't wear yellow or neutrals.

Busted: If a redhead is going to wear yellow, we always encourage a burnt yellow. You can also incorporate yellow jeans, shoes or pants as an accessory.

4. *Myth:* Redheads should not wear green. Many people say this, especially redheads themselves because they feel red hair and green is too Christmassy and/or leprechaun-like.

Busted: Green is by far the best color for a redhead. But again, it's all about the tone.

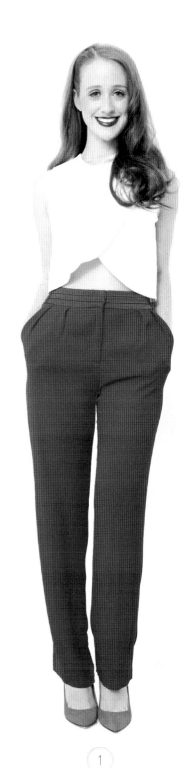

1

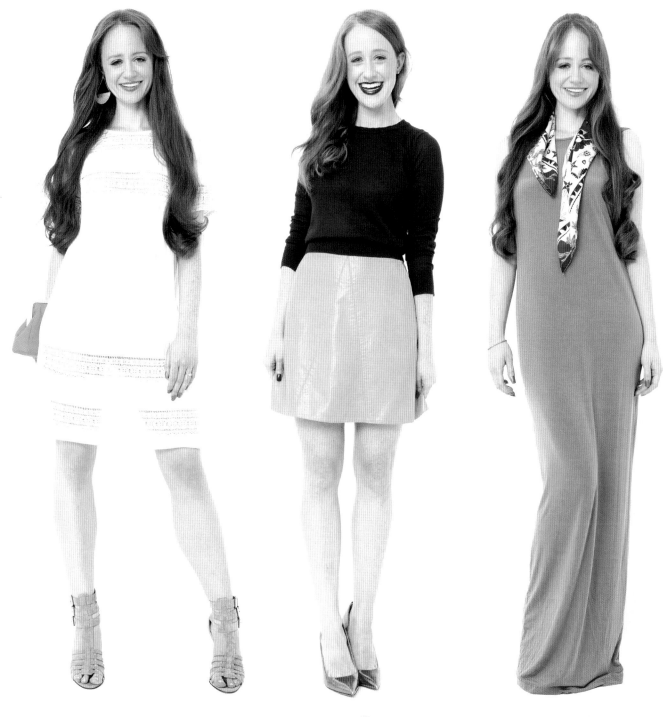

Always remember, you're amazing! Each and every day, *Rock it like a Redhead!*

Have questions or want further beauty tips?
Tweet us using #H2BARBook

acknowledgments

We want to thank our parents, Michael and Jan, for always pushing us to think big. If it were not for your support, we would not have strived for our dreams. We love you.

To our family, especially Kathleen Demoe, Mary Phelan, Lucio and Rosemary Vendetti.

To our husbands, Joshua Hodges and Brian Thomas. We feel blessed to have married our best friends. Thank you for your support and love.

To Kiera Doyle, our hairstylist, and Andrew Reynolds, our wardrobe stylist. We are so lucky to have met you both in high school and thank you for believing in us from the start. You're both incredibly talented, and we are so thankful to have you in our lives.

To everyone who made this book possible:

+ Luciana Pampalone, photographer

+ Flynn Marie Pyykkonen, makeup artist

+ RPZL Hair Extension & Blowout Bar

+ EVA New York

+ The Lash Loft NYC

+ Nicole Miller

+ Blo Blow Dry Bar

+ CHI Farouk Systems

+ AMIKA

And thank you to all who contributed tips, suggestions and quotes for this book.

And, finally, to Page Street Publishing and our literary agent, Rachel Vogel. Thank you for seeing and believing in our vision.

about the authors

Adrienne and Stephanie Vendetti are sisters and cofounders of the brand How to be a Redhead. Its mission is to empower every redhead woman to feel confident, look amazing and to rock her beauty. Red hair is more than a color, *it's a lifestyle!*

The sisters were born as natural redheads and struggled to find beauty and fashion items that catered to trendy redheaded women. Since there was no place for them to turn to for advice, they created HowtoBeaRedhead.com for redheads throughout the world. Since its launch, it has been recognized by top companies and press in the world, and in 2012, Adrienne and Stephanie became L'Oreal Paris Brand Ambassadors. HowtoBeaRedhead. com also been mentioned in outlets such as the *New York Times*, ABC News, *SHAPE* magazine, Refinery29 and many others.

The Vendetti sisters are now known as the redhead spokeswomen of the world and regularly hear from their fans that they love How to be a Redhead for what it stands for as much as for what it offers—gaining confidence and overcoming adversity.

How to Be a Redhead is based in New York, NY. Adrienne lives in Wilmington, NC, with her (redhead) husband, Josh, and their two basset hounds, Jack and Sam. Stephanie lives in Charlotte, NC (where How to be a Redhead's second office is located) with her husband, Brian. The sisters love traveling across the United States and world for their red-carpet beauty events called *Rock it Like a Redhead*. It's rare that you will not find the sisters together or without rocking their favorite beauty item: mascara. And if you're wondering, they are not twins!

index